The National Study of Health and Growth

The National Study of Health and Growth

Roberto J. Rona and Susan Chinn

Department of Public Health Sciences
King's College, London

with contributions from
Walter W. Holland,
James M. Tanner,
and
Peter G. J. Burney

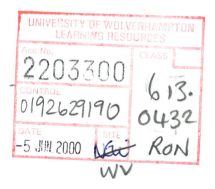
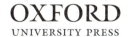

OXFORD
UNIVERSITY PRESS

OXFORD

UNIVERSITY PRESS

Great Clarendon Street, Oxford OX2 6DP

Oxford University Press is a department of the University of Oxford.
It furthers the University's objective of excellence in research, scholarship,
and education by publishing worldwide in

Oxford New York

Athens Auckland Bangkok Bogotá Buenos Aires Calcutta
Cape Town Chennai Dar es Salaam Delhi Florence Hong Kong Istanbul
Karachi Kuala Lumpur Madrid Melbourne Mexico City Mumbai
Nairobi Paris São Paulo Singapore Taipei Tokyo Toronto Warsaw

and associated companies in Berlin Ibadan

Oxford is a registered trade mark of Oxford University Press
in the UK and in certain other countries

Published in the United States
by Oxford University Press Inc., New York

A catalogue record for this book is available from the British Library

Library of Congress Cataloging in Publication Data

Rona, Roberto J.
National study of health and growth / Roberto J. Rona and Susan
Chinn ; with contributions from Walter W. Holland, James M. Tanner,
and Peter G.J. Burney.
Includes bibliographical references and index.
1. Children–Great Britain–Growth Longitudinal studies.
2. Children–Health and hygiene–Great Britain Longitudinal studies.
I. Chinn, Susan. II. Title.
RJ131.R637   1999   614.4'241'083–dc21   99–14303
ISBN 0 19 262919 0
1 3 5 7 9 10 8 6 4 2

Typeset by Bibliocraft, Dundee
Printed in Great Britain
on acid-free paper by
Bookcraft (Bath) Ltd.
Midsomer Norton, Avon

Foreword

This volume will take its place on my bookshelf along with the four great classic works on human macronutrient nutrition. Benedict *et al.* (1919) and Keys *et al.* (1950) reported studies on semi-starved volunteers, in order to understand the physiology of severe malnutrition which was rife in Europe after the First and Second World War respectively. Sims *et al.* (1968) studied volunteers who were overfed, in order to find out if the insulin insensitivity which is associated with obesity is *caused* by the obesity, and showed that it was. Stein *et al.* (1975) traced the consequences up to 30 years later of the famine which affected north-west Holland in 1944–45. These are classic never-to-be-repeated studies on which much of our present understanding of the effects of human under- or over-nutrition is based. They will not be repeated because in the current climate of funding, and the ethics of human research, the experiments would not be approved. The Dutch famine was a result of a war-time situation which everyone hopes will not recur.

I think the *National Study of Health and Growth* (NSHG) will achieve recognition as a classic of stature comparable to those mentioned above. It will not be repeated, because the circumstances which initiated it are unlikely to recur, and because the question it was set up to answer would no longer be tackled by serial measurements of the height of school children. Three decades ago the scientists who advised the government in the UK on human nutrition had served their apprenticeship in third-world countries, where slowing of height gain in children was the most sensitive and reliable evidence of undernutrition. Professor Tanner was the guru of anthopometry. The experts believed that if children over the age of seven years suffered nutritionally by being deprived of free school milk this would be best detected by slowing of·height gain.

What actually happened to height velocity you can learn by reading the pages which follow, but that is not the reason why this volume is so significant. As the NSHG went on, the old generation of nutritionists (in which I include myself) learned a lot about the variables other than height velocity which are relevant to nutritional status in children in affluent countries. We no longer accept that a child's nutrition is correct because it is travelling along an appropriate centile of height-for-age. During the 23 year life-span of the NSHG many things changed: the development of new computing and statistical techniques, the shift in employment and ethnic structure in the UK, the recognition of cigarette smoking as a public health hazard, the replacement of undernutrition by obesity as the most prevalent nutritional disorder among both children and adults. With these changes the mighty juggernaut of the NSHG had to adapt to address these new problems, while retaining the tremendous power of long-term serial measurements. Roberto Rona and Susan Chinn have made a selection of some findings from this unique study for inclusion in this volume. I predict that many generations to come of nutritionists and social scientists will continue to delve into the data in this book, and into those archived at the University of Essex, just as we still delve into the data of Benedict, Keys, Sims and Stein.

J. S. Garrow

References

Benedict, F. G., Miles, W. R., Roth, P., Smith, M. (1919). *Human vitality and efficiency under prolonged restricted diet*, pp. 83. Washington, DC: Carnegie Institution publ. 280.

Keys, A., Brozek, J., Hanschel, A., Mickelson, O., Taylor, H. L. (1950). *The biology of human starvation*, pp. 1385. University of Minnesota Press, Minneapolis.

Sims, E. A. H., Goldman, R. F., Gluck C. M., Horton, E. S., Kelleher, P. C., Rowe, D. W. (1968). Experimental obesity in man. *Transactions of the Association of American Physicians*, **81**: 153–70.

Stein, Z., Susser, M., Saenger, G., Marolla, F. (1975). *Famine and human development: the Dutch winter hunger of 1944–1945*, pp. 284. Oxford University Press, New York.

Preface

The National Study of Health and Growth (NSHG) studied English and Scottish children aged 5–11 years from 1972 to 1994, a period which saw great changes in health and welfare provision and social circumstances in Britain. The study was unique in its continuity of data for 23 years, providing information on trends in height, weight-for-height, subcutaneous arm tissue, and asthma, as well as a wealth of information on risk factors for impaired growth, the impact of changes in welfare policy, and the distribution of coronary heart disease risk factors in children. The contribution of the study extended to topics including nocturnal enuresis, disturbed sleep, food intolerance, and passive smoking. The primary schools originally sampled in 1972 provided cross-sections of mainly white English and Scottish children, around 9000 a year in total. The addition of inner-city schools from 1983 onwards enabled a comparison to be made of the attained growth of ethnic minority groups with white children living in similar conditions, and with the general population, and, uniquely, of trends in growth. Over the 23 years 87 424 children were eligible to take part in the study at least once, with a total of 172 790 records. The data are being archived with The Data Archive at the University of Essex.

With such diversity of information the publications from the study, now over 100 in number, are distributed across a large number of general medical, epidemiological, paediatric, and anthropological journals. This book brings together the various findings in the changing context of the study, providing an overview and assessment of the contribution of the study, which is only possible now that data collection has ceased. The book does not attempt to summarize every finding. Inevitably, from a study lasting over 20 years, some of the findings are no longer topical and some have been superseded. However, some of the insights that are given into conducting this complex study are not published elsewhere.

This book will be of prime interest to researchers in child health and nutrition, and to specialists in growth and respiratory illness, and of general interest to anyone mounting a study of schoolchildren. A number of topics will be relevant to consultants in paediatric subspecialties, such as endocrinology, and others to researchers in respiratory medicine. It will also be important for physical anthropologists and nutritionists. It is not aimed at undergraduates, but may be helpful for those developing a paediatric or nutrition project. Finally, statisticians in the field are not forgotten. The study took place over a period during which enormous changes in statistical methodology and computing took place. While technical details are kept to a minimum the issues that the design of the study presented for the analysis of the data are summarized, and the implications of changing methodology are discussed.

The main authors were the project leader and statistician, from 1976 and 1977 onwards, respectively.

London   R.J.R.
March 1999   S.C.

Acknowledgements

This book is based on our perceptions of what were the important contributions, the main achievements, and the lessons learnt from a study that was carried out over nearly a quarter of a century. We take full responsibility for the final product. However, we would not have been able to write this book without the contribution to the NSHG of so many colleagues and friends who were members of the team. We have pleasure and trepidation in taking the opportunity to thank those who made possible the success of the study—pleasure in giving recognition to our colleagues who shared our responsibility, and trepidation because in our attempt to achieve fairness we may have forgotten or wrongly omitted some names from the long list of team members. We plead for forgiveness.

We are indebted to Professor Walter W. Holland who continuously supported the study and helped us to solve difficult problems at the interface with the Department of Health, Health Authorities, and Education Authorities, and to Professor P. G. J. Burney who succeeded him as head of department. We thank Professors Lesley Irwig and Doug Altman and Dr Judith Cook who mounted and managed this extensive study in its first 5 years. We are full of admiration for their achievement. Professor Charles du V. Florey was the adviser to the team until the beginning of the 1980s, to which he brought great intellectual rigour.

We wish to acknowledge the friendly and constant support to the NSHG of Professors James M. Tanner and John Garrow. Professor Tanner was an authoritative disseminator of our work. Professor John Garrow, as chairman of the Sub-committee on Nutritional Surveillance of the Department of Health, always gave constructive and encouraging hearing to our reports to the Sub-committee.

Many colleagues carried out analyses based on NSHG data, were co-authors, commented on early drafts of our papers, or were responsible for piloting new measurements for the study. We especially thank Drs Jane Melia, Charles Price, Martin Gulliford, Judith Hammond, Enric Duran-Tauleria, Richard Morris, Miss Alison Smith, Mr John Hughes, and Mrs Leah Li for their contributions.

Mrs Juliana Oladuti is praised without being named in Chapter 3. Without her efficient administration the task of managing the study would have been extremely difficult. She was also invaluable for bringing to our attention problems within the team that needed prompt and fair resolution. Miss Sheena Somerville was the longest serving fieldworker. We are grateful for her dedication and persistence in bringing inconsistencies to our attention.

Over 23 years the study had 32 fieldworkers, at least 25 assistant statisticians, and 12 secretaries. They were invaluable in their contributions to the study. We have resisted the temptation to name every one and feel it unfair to select only some for praise. The study would have been impossible without their dedicated work.

We are also grateful to our helpers in the 56 areas of the study, the headteachers and their staff, nurses, doctors, and administrators. Without them the NSHG would not have happened nor, of most importance, without the participation of 87 000 children and their parents or guardians.

The study was funded by the Department of Health and Scottish Home and Health Department.

Roberto J. Rona and Susan Chinn

Contents

1 Background to the study

Introduction

In 1970, amongst other proposals on changes in welfare, the then UK Government with Margaret Thatcher as Secretary of State for Education announced its intention of discontinuing free school milk for children over seven years of age. This led to protests with banner headlines of 'Margaret Thatcher, milk snatcher'. As a result an undertaking was given that 'the nutritional status of the population would be carefully monitored with a view to detecting any unforeseen adverse effects which might arise from the change at a stage when they were mild and reversible' (Department of Health and Social Security 1973). The National Study of Health and Growth was set up as part of the fulfilment of this undertaking. It began in 1972 and continued for 23 years.

Historical perspective

The relationship between the growth of children and their socioeconomic background had been extensively studied. Bransby *et al.* (1946) and the Oxford Child Health Survey (Acheson and Hewitt 1954) had shown that children from poor homes or large families were consistently smaller and lighter than those from wealthy homes or smaller families. The association between height and weight and whether the mother worked or not had previously been observed during World War II. Two possible explanations were advanced: if the mother worked she would eat in the works canteen and thus more food was available for the child, or that the family was better off financially.

An investigation of the effects of environmental and personal factors on respiratory symptoms and ventilatory function, among 10 971 schoolchildren in Kent in 1964 and 1965 (Holland *et al.* 1969), provided data for a study of the influence of some environmental factors on the heights and weights of children. This study examined three factors: father's social class; the number of siblings; and the number of hours for which the mother was employed. Weight was found to be associated with all three factors in both sexes in at least one age group. No association was found between weight for height and social class, but was shown for the other two factors; body mass index declined with the number of siblings and increased with number of hours worked by the mother, and the associations were greater in the oldest (14–17 years) than in the youngest (5–8 years) children (Topp *et al.* 1970).

That growth rate and quality of nutrition were related had been established in a number of surveys (e.g. Howe and Schiller 1952; Widdowson 1951; Widdowson and McCance 1954). In view of the above findings, and the interest at that time of Kent County Council Health Department and the Department of Health and Social Security in the standards of nutrition among schoolchildren, further investigations were undertaken between 1968 and 1970 to examine the dietary intake of schoolchildren and its relationship to health and socioeconomic factors, and to determine the nature and extent of poor nutrition. Data from three sources were used, a one-week weighed diet record, a comprehensive socioeconomic questionnaire, and a medical examination. Approximately 800 primary and secondary schoolchildren were included in the study (J. Cook *et al.* 1973; Topp *et al.* 1972). This study showed that those who drank school milk had a greater intake of energy and nutrients than those who did not, but this was not related to height, weight, or obesity (J. Cook *et al.*

1975*a*). The children who took school meals had a higher lunch-time intake of nutrients. Children from larger families and fatherless children were more likely to take school meals (J. Cook *et al.* 1975*b*), and these groups and lower social class children obtained a higher proportion of their intake of nutrients from lunch than other children. The children from one-child households had significantly higher intakes of most nutrients than other children and were more likely to be obese (Jacoby *et al.* 1975). The level of the household's disposable income was not related to nutrient intake. The clinical examination revealed no evidence of undernutrition; nearly 11% were classified as obese.

These studies serve as background to the involvement of St Thomas' Hospital Medical School, London, in the NSHG (National Study of Health and Growth). When the Government decided to change its policy for the provision of free school meals and welfare it was considered that standards of living, income, nutrition, etc. had greatly improved since the end of World War II. There was no overt evidence of undernutrition in schoolchildren, as shown by the absence of reports of rickets or other nutritional deficiency conditions.

The birth of the National Study of Health and Growth

In October 1970 the Government, in a White Paper 'New Policies for Public Spending', announced changes in the arrangements for the provision of welfare milk, school milk, and school meals. School meals were to rise to 12p, shortly after to 14p, with the ultimate objective that school meals would not be subsidized, with the exceptions of households where there was a defined level of hardship. The White Paper also announced the intention to discontinue the free supply of a third of a pint of milk to each pupil after the end of the summer term following his or her seventh birthday. This major change in welfare policy was opposed by many groups. Those concerned with health in general supported the change, but with the proviso that: provision should be made for those considered to be at highest risk; the system would enable adverse changes in growth, nutrition, and health to be identified while they were still mild; and areas and populations put at risk by any such changes would be identified (Department of Health and Social Security 1973).

After a great deal of discussion it was decided that the lessons learned in the studies of Kent schoolchildren should be applied on a national scale. The Kent Nutrition Study had demonstrated that although a weighed, dietary intake study could be used in schoolchildren, it was both expensive and time-consuming and that reporting of results was delayed. It was thus difficult to envisage using such a method on a national scale with enough children in each social-class and age–sex group to provide findings sufficiently robust to influence policy. A COMA (Committee on Medical Aspects of Food Policy) Sub-committee on nutritional surveillance was formed to consider arrangements required for the prediction and assessment of any nutritional effects of changes in welfare policy.

In its first report the COMA Sub-committee argued that school meals and milk were intended to make a substantial contribution to the nutrient intake of children (Department of Health and Social Security 1973). While children whose parents were deemed unable to replace the State provision would be provided with a similar level of dietary support as before the changes, there were uncertainties as to whether other parents would fill the vacuum left by the State. Thus either the diet provided by parents would be insufficient, and as a consequence the nutritional status of children would suffer, or the food provided by parents would be of higher energy content and this would increase the prevalence of obesity. The latter was unlikely to occur given the already high fat content of school meals reported in most dietary surveys (J. Cook *et al.* 1975*b*; Darke *et al.* 1980; Department of Health 1989).

It was logical that the COMA Sub-comittee recommended the assessment of growth, especially height, as the main measure of nutritional status. Weight was considered a secondary measure as it was thought too sensitive to transient changes. The Sub-comittee favoured the measurement of rate of growth as the most sensitive indicator for assessing nutritional status. However, in Chapter 4 it is explained why attained height rather than rate of growth was monitored in the population. The Sub-comittee was not in favour of assessing dietary deficiency by looking for signs of malnutrition or assessing biochemical indices.

The Sub-comittee proposed, among other studies, to set up a monitoring system of children between 5 and 11 years of age. Records of height and weight were to be obtained each year so that growth increments according to age could be assessed. In parallel to the primary school monitoring system a preschool system was also proposed. The Sub-comittee was ambiguous about the value of measuring skinfold thickness.

The Social Medicine and Health Services Research Unit in the Department of Clinical Epidemiology and Social Medicine at St. Thomas' Hospital Medical School was given responsibility for the primary school monitoring system, initially for a period of five years from 1972, and the Department of Human Nutrition, London School of Hygiene and Tropical Medicine, was commissioned to undertake a preschool study for the same length of time. The stated aim of the NSHG (Department of Health and Social Security 1973) was to 'set up an anthropometric system of surveillance on selected growth, nutritional and health characteristics which may help to identify the effects of changes in food policy while any such effects are reversible'. It was not foreseen that the NSHG would run for 23 years, with final data collection being made in 1994.

The organizers of the monitoring system favoured the following characteristics for the study: that measurements should be very few and simple; and only basic dietary, health, and socio-economic data should be included in a questionnaire posted to parents. The measurements chosen by the organizers were height, weight, and triceps skinfold thickness. Individual questions were kept simple, but the temptation to collect a considerable amount of information was less well resisted, as detailed in Chapter 2. The Sub-comittee on Nutritional Surveillance was non-committal on the value of measuring skinfold thickness in the NSHG. However, results from several studies have shown that skinfold thickness is a more sensitive measure of increases in fatness than weight-for-height (Chinn and Rona 1987a; Gortmaker et al. 1987; Harlan et al. 1988; Hughes et al. 1997). With hindsight it would have been helpful for the NSHG to have measured not only triceps skinfold thickness but also subscapular skinfold thickness, as fat distribution was later found to be related to coronary heart disease (Lapidus et al. 1984).

There was a commitment to collect information on sociodemographic characteristics related to nutrition as it was recognized that the population at greatest risk from the changes in policy would be those living in poor social conditions (Department of Health and Social Security 1973). The plan was to collect information on an annual basis in 5–10-year-old children attending the same schools. Geographical areas were chosen by stratified random sampling weighted towards the poorer end of the distribution, as described in Chapter 2. Schools were chosen within areas by the health and education authorities. Results were therefore not truly representative of the population from a strict statistical view.

At the outset the organizers made it clear that one of the limitations of the study was the lack of dietary information. It is difficult for those who have recently started research on nutritional epidemiology to understand why it was not possible to include a simpler method than the one-week weighed dietary record, for example a food frequency questionnaire (Nelson and Bingham 1997; Willetts 1990), but at that time nutritionists were critical of the use of any methodology other than the one-week dietary record. Marr (1971) provided a lucid account of the conflicting views on suitable methods for dietary surveys at the time. Professor Angus Thompson, who became the second chairman of the Sub-comittee on Nutritional Surveillance, was of the view that it was preferable to have a high accuracy of dietary information in a small sample than unmeasured quantities of food from every subject in a study. Mann and colleagues, who had participated in the Framingham study in the USA, were of the opinion that the success of epidemiological studies was critically dependent upon the completeness of response of the sample (Mann *et al.* 1962). Marr's view of the simplified methods of dietary information was that their epidemiological value had yet to be proven. Thus the use of an alternative method to the one-week weighed record would have lacked credibility in the British academic and policy community at that time.

No other limitations were identified at the outset of the study. However, about 16 years later officers of the Department of Health felt that a representative sample would be preferable to the chosen design of the NSHG. By then we were reluctant to change the design of the NSHG because it would have limited its main value, which was to allow unbiased comparisons over time on growth and other measurements. Chapter 2 discusses the advantages and disadvantages of the chosen design for its main purpose and subsidiary aims.

2 Design, data collection, and analysis

Introduction

The NSHG, designed in 1970 and 1971 as a 5-year study, started in 1972 but continued until 1994. It is hard to appreciate the changes that have taken place in methodology for the design and execution of studies over this 23-year period. In 1972 punched cards had only recently replaced paper tape as the standard input medium for computers, but many people reading this book will have used neither. A multiple regression analysis on data for one year of the study had to be carried out remotely on a 'large' university mainframe machine, and one was lucky to run more than two such analyses in one day, while now several years' data can be analysed in seconds on a personal computer. This chapter should be read with such advances in mind.

Study design

The study was conceived with a mixed longitudinal design (Fig. 2.1). The children sampled in any one year were a cross-section of the population, but there was also a longitudinal element as schools

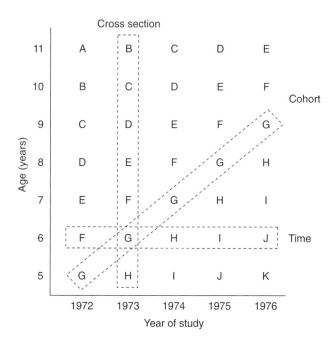

Fig. 2.1 Design of the NSHG from 1972 to 1976.

were revisited and the children were eligible for as long as they attended the chosen schools and were of primary school age. The rationale was that this would allow differences in growth to be analysed over time between children of the same age, between groups cross-sectionally, and with age in a given cohort (Department of Health and Social Security 1973; Irwig 1976).

Initial sampling

The Sub-committee on Nutritional Surveillance decided that the NSHG sample should be weighted to overselect 'poorer' children, as these would be more vulnerable to any adverse social or environmental change. For administrative reasons it was decided to select complete primary schools, rather than individual children, and to weight the sample by a stratified selection of areas. Limited data were available on which to base the stratification, as the study was designed before the 1971 census data were available. The percentage of economically active people who were unemployed in August 1970 was obtained for each employment exchange area in England and Scotland. The Department of Education and Science supplied the percentage uptake of free school meals for autumn 1969 (England) and January 1969 (Scotland) and the percentage of school leavers at the minimum age for 1970 and 1969, respectively, for each LEA (Local Education Authority). The data for LEAs were then ascribed to employment exchange areas, with weighting for split employment exchange areas as appropriate (Altman, unpublished paper). The three variables were combined into indices of socioeconomic status for England and Scotland separately, and the indices divided into six strata for England and four for Scotland. Employment exchange areas were then selected from strata with weighting towards the poorer strata (Irwig 1976). A total of 22 areas in England and 6 in Scotland were chosen.

Within each area, medical and educational personnel were asked to select a primary school or schools 'representative of their area classification' to provide a total of at least 300 pupils (Irwig 1976). Hence sampling of schools was not random and, with two of the variables used to construct the index being derived for employment exchange areas from the larger LEAs, there was considerable potential for the desired weighting towards 'poorer' children not being realized. The English NSHG social class distribution was found to be close to that found at the 1971 census for England and Wales (Rona and Altman 1977). Although not strictly representative from a sampling point of view, the sample has often been referred to as representative, particularly to distinguish the original sample from the inner-city sample added later.

Main phases of the study

Although conceived as a 5-year study (Irwig 1976), the full implications of the mixed longitudinal design were not appreciated at the outset. The questionnaire sent to all parents in 1972 was designed to collect data for children entering the study. Questions such as those on attacks of respiratory illness referred to the child's lifetime experience. This was not appropriate for children who were being followed-up, so a separate questionnaire with questions referring to the last 12 months was used for children followed-up in 1973, and the dual system continued until 1976. The consequence of this was that from 1973 to 1976 some items of data, viewed cross-sectionally, were not entirely compatible. This inevitably caused a number of difficulties for data checking and analysis. The opportunity was also taken in 1973 to modify the data collection form for the measurements in the light of the experience of the 1972 survey, so that even for new entrants some data were not entirely compatible between 1972 and 1973 to 1976.

Enthusiasm, and input from several disciplines, led to a fairly lengthy questionnaire. This may have contributed to the decision to provide a shorter questionnaire, with questions particular to the child only, for children with an older sibling also in the NSHG. Family data then needed to be transferred between siblings, but this relied on an accurate family list being provided by the school. This system was used for 1972, and for follow-up children, but not new entrants, from 1973 to 1976.

A change of project leader in 1976 combined with funding being granted for a further 5 years prompted a rethink, to the other extreme. A simplified questionnaire was introduced for all children; this meant that cross-sectional analyses were straightforward, but items such as birth-weight were unnecessarily collected more than once for most children and that household questions were answered for each child in the family. Funding of a third phase prompted a second rethink, and the design of separate, but compatible, questionnaires for new entrant and follow-up children. The new entrant questionnaire was used for all children in 1982 and 1983 so that comparable data were obtained on birthweight and other items that needed to be obtained once only. These questionnaires were used, with minor modifications, until the end of the study in 1994.

Inner-city areas

The third phase of the study ran from 1982 to 1994. The change to the questionnaire has already been outlined above, but there was an even more fundamental change. It had been recognized for some time that not only did the selection of schools not achieve the weighting towards poorer children that had been thought desirable, but that inner-city areas, and ethnic minority children in particular, were too few to allow any useful comparison. In order to include a sample of such areas and children, but at the same time preserve the existing monitoring system, a 2-year cycle was introduced. The existing areas were visited in even years, and 20 English inner-city areas were surveyed each odd year from 1983 to 1993. The opportunity was taken to increase the Scottish sample, which had also proved rather small for drawing useful conclusions, from 6 to 14 areas.

The inner-city areas were selected during 1982 using the small area statistics from the 1971 census, as data from the 1981 census were not then available. There were five items extracted manually from the microfiche for each ward of the County and London Boroughs: the percentage of economically active men unemployed but seeking employment; the percentage of households with exclusive use of all basic amenities; the percentage of households with more than 1.5 persons per room; the percentage of persons born in New Commonwealth America; and the percentage of persons born in New Commonwealth Asia. Ten 'inner-city' wards were chosen with extremely high values of the first or third items, or extremely low values of the second. Using the last two items of data, as proxies for a high percentage of Black or Indian subcontinent origin residents, five wards with the highest values of each were chosen.

Wards with a high proportion of ethnic minority residents also tended to display characteristics of inner-city areas, so all 20 areas are referred to as inner city. The education authority for each borough was asked to identify the school for which the catchment area was most central to the ward, and also asked whether any substantial redevelopment had taken place since 1971. Of the first 20 areas selected, 16 agreed to co-operate, and the remaining 4 were replaced by the next most extreme on the selection variable(s).

Replacement of areas

The same 30 schools and 28 areas took part for the first 5 years of the study. As will be discussed in Chapter 3 this required considerable commitment, and having been told in 1972 that the NSHG would last for 5 years a few declined to take part in 1977. One area in Glasgow was so redeveloped that there was no alternative to its replacement. When the health and education authorities were able and willing to continue to participate, selection of an alternative school in the same area was the first option. If this was not possible a new area was chosen from the same sampling stratum. The changes that took place in the representative sample are summarized in Table 2.1. At the beginning of the third phase two areas declined to participate further, but as can be seen the NSHG was very

Table 2.1 Number of changes in areas and schools in the representative samples

Year	Number of changes in area	Number of changes in schools		
		Replacement	Addition	Loss
Phase 1				
1972–76	—	—	—	—
Phase 2				
1977	5[1]	3	—	—
1978–79	—	—	—	—
1980–81	—	—	—	1[2]
Phase 3				
1982[3]	2	1	1[2]	—
1983[4]	—	—	—	—
1984	2	—	—	1[5]
1985–87	—	—	—	—
1988	1	1	1	—
1989	1	—	—	—
1990	—	1	—	—
1991	—	—	—	—
1992	1	1	—	—
1993	—	1	—	—
1994	1[6]	—	—	—

[1]One replacement area agreed too late to take part in 1977, and joined in 1978.
[2]In one area a replacement school was not recruited until 1982.
[3]One Scottish area transferred from even- to odd-year participation.
[4]Representative sample in odd years from 1983 onwards consisted of one existing area[3] and eight new Scottish areas.
[5]Loss of one school within an area in which several small schools were recruited.
[6]One area declined to take part in 1994 and was not replaced for the final year of the study.

successful in maintaining participation. The net result was that 12 of the original 22 English areas, and two of the original six Scottish areas, took part with no change of school over the whole period, a total of 17 surveys. Of the extra eight Scottish areas, six from 1983 were unchanged for their six surveys. No inner-city area was replaced; one school was replaced within the same ward in 1985, and another in 1991.

Response rates

For the purposes of studying trends over time the non-random selection of schools was not disadvantageous. It was necessary to gain the co-operation of the education and health authorities not only to mount the study but to achieve a high response rate, and in this respect too the study was highly successful. The response to measurement was around 98% in the representative samples in the first 10 years, dropping to around 95% at the end of the study. However the last 3-years' response rates were influenced by the need to obtain positive consent for a fingerprick test in 1992 and 1993 and venepuncture in 1994 for one age group. Response to the questionnaire self-administered by the parents fluctuated, there appearing to be some fatigue towards the end of each

Table 2.2 Numbers of children eligible and response rates in the English and Scottish representative samples

Year	Total eligible	Response to measurement (%)	Response to questionnaire (%)
1972	10 543	98.9	90.2
1973	10 683	98.5	89.3
1974	10 632	97.7	84.4
1975	10 414	97.9	84.4
1976	10 351	98.0	80.3
1977	9923	98.4	90.7
1978	9996	98.3	89.7
1979	9720	98.0	89.7
1980	8750	97.8	88.3
1981	8245	97.8	87.3
1982	8118	96.8	87.8
1983[1]	2851	96.0	90.2
1984	8109	97.2	89.9
1985	2595	96.4	95.8
1986	8007	97.7	91.4
1987	2593	97.8	96.5
1988	8617	97.9	92.9
1989	2552	96.9	96.4
1990	8499	96.6	92.3
1991	2527	97.8	96.5
1992	8294	94.3	92.4
1993	2514	95.8	94.9
1994	8257	94.2	91.6

[1]From 1983 only nine areas, in the Scottish representative sample, were surveyed in odd years.

phase. Numbers of eligible children and the response rates are shown in Tables 2.2 and 2.3. Response to measurement, and to the questionnaire, was lower in the inner-city sample than in the representative samples, but still high, and response in the Scottish sample was slightly higher than in the English representative sample. The response rates are for the return of the questionnaire with at least one question answered. Response rates for individual questions, particularly those relating to social class, were lower.

Data collection

Throughout, there were core items of data collected, both measurements and questionnaire items answered by parents or guardians, as well as additional items—some of which lasted for the whole of a main phase, and others which were added in a specific year or years. These are summarized in Tables 2.4 to 2.6. The lists are not exhaustive; a few measurements or questions that have not been used in any analyses have been omitted. Because the main aim of the study was to monitor changes over time, as far as possible no changes were made to the methods of measurement or wording of questions. However, particularly for the latter, alterations were necessary at times, either because it

Table 2.3 Numbers of children eligible and response rates in the inner-city sample

Year	Total eligible	Response to measurement (%)	Response to questionnaire (%)
1983	7459	94.6	82.8
1985	7348	94.8	83.2
1987	7320	95.9	83.5
1989	7271	94.3	78.0
1991	7462	95.5	81.5
1993	7447	90.9	78.7

Table 2.4 Years of collection of anthropometric and other measurements, and other data recorded at the time of fieldwork

	Year	Age group (years)
Core measurements		
Height	1972–1994	4–11
Weight	1972–1994	4–11
Triceps skinfold thickness	1972–1994	4–11
Subscapular skinfold thickness	1989–1994	4–11
Other measurements		
Lung function (FVC, FEV_1, FEF_{25-75}, FEF_{75-85})	1987–1990	7–11
'Rising-nine' children only		
Biceps skinfold thickness	1992–1994	8–9
Suprailiac skinfold thickness	1992–1994	8–9
Systolic and diastolic blood pressure	1992–1994	8–9
Arm circumference	1994	8–9
Serum total cholesterol (fingerprick test)	1992–1993	8–9
Fitness (cycle ergometer test)	1992–1993	8–9
Bronchial responsiveness (exercise challenge)	1992–1993	8–9
Serum total and HDL cholesterol, ferritin, and haematology (venous sample)	1994	8–9
Other data obtained during fieldwork		
Date of birth	1972–1994	4–11
Sex of child	1972–1994	4–11
Date of measurement	1972–1994	4–11
Ethnic origin	1972–1994	4–11
Language spoken at home	1983, 1985, 1987, 1989, 1991, 1993	4–11

became clear that the question had been misunderstood, because of socioeconomic changes creating a need to collect extra data, for example on long-term unemployment, or because terminology had changed, for example in relation to receipt of benefits.

Items are considered as 'core' if collected throughout, or, if once introduced or reintroduced, they continued for the length of the study and were unlikely to have been dropped had the study continued further. For both measurements and questionnaire items there was a balance that had to be reached between data that would be useful if collected, but were not absolutely essential to the

Table 2.5   Core questionnaire items (all children)

Birthweight (N)	1972–1994
School meal provision (N, F)	1972–1994
School milk provision (N, F)	1972–1994
Number of older siblings (N, F)	1972–1994
Number of younger siblings (N, F)	1972–1981
Total number of siblings	1977–1994
Number of rooms in home (F)	1973–1976, 1982–1994
Number of people in household (N, F)	1972–1994
Mother's height (N)	1972–1994
Mother's weight (N)	1972–1976, 1982–1994
Father's height (N)	1972–1994
Father's weight (N)	1972–1976, 1982–1994
Mother's education (N)	1972–1994
Father's education (N)	1972–1976, 1989–1994
Mother's employment/social class (N, F)[1]	1972–1976 (1977–1981), 1982–1994
Father's employment/social class (N, F)	1972–1994
One-parent family	1977–1994
Receipt of benefits (N, F)	1972–1994
Mother's hours of work outside home	1982–1994
Attacks of bronchitis (N, F)	1972–1994
Attacks of pneumonia (N, F)	1972–1981
Attacks of asthma (F)	1973–1994
Respiratory symptoms	1973–1977, 1982–1994
Passive smoking	1977, 1982, 1987–1994
Length of gestation of child	1977–1994

N: Included in new entrant questionnaire when applicable 1972–1994.
F: Included in follow-up questionnaire 1973–1976.
[1]1977–1981 only for single-parent mothers.

Table 2.6   Occasional questionnaire topics (all children)

Household cooking fuel (F)	1973–1977, 1987
Household heating fuel (F)	1973–1977, 1987
Parental assessment of school meals	1981
Child a vegetarian	1983–1994
Food intolerance	1984
Time child sleeps at night	1988
Parents' atopic diseases	1989–1991
Medication for chest illness	1990–1991
Disturbed sleep and enuresis	1991–1992
Frequency items of food intake	1992–1994
Family history of heart attacks	1992–1994

study, and keeping the fieldwork and questionnaire to a length compatible with a good response from schools and parents. Thus some items of data were collected for selected years or age groups for research that was topical, or required only a cross-sectional sample and not longitudinal data. The simplification of the questionnaire in 1977 led to items considered non-essential at that time to be dropped, or included only as extra items in 1977. However, a number of these, notably respiratory symptoms and parents' reported weights, were reintroduced in 1982.

Measurements

Height, weight, and triceps skinfold thickness were measured for all children throughout, and subscapular skinfold added in 1989 after distribution of fat became an issue (Lapidus *et al.* 1984). The two other skinfold measurements, at the biceps and suprailiac sites, were included for 'rising-nine' children in 1992 to 1994 in order to assess fatness more fully, along with other cardiovascular risk factors, in these years. Measurements were made during one week in each area on school premises. The child's gender, date of birth, ethnic origin as assessed by the fieldworker, and the date of measurement were recorded for all children. Absentees were measured on return to the school if possible. As far as possible the week scheduled for each area stayed the same from year to year so that children were measured approximately annually.

Height

Height was measured on a specially designed Holtain stadiometer, using the method recommended by Tanner *et al.* (1966). The child was stretched gently, with the head kept in the Frankfort plane and the heels checked to make sure they remained on the ground. From 1972 to 1976, the stadiometer scale was read to the last complete 0.5 cm, but to the last 0.1 cm from 1977 onwards. In comparisons over time, 0.25 cm or 0.05 cm was added to the measurements as appropriate to correct the bias. From 1972 to 1976 a clerk stretched the child while a school nurse read the measurement scale. As correct stretching of the child is the biggest determinant of accuracy this was changed, so that from 1977 onwards the fieldworker stretched while the nurse read the scale. In this case the desirability of the latter procedure outweighed the criterion of comparability over time.

Weight

Children were weighed in underpants, with their weight recorded to the last complete 100 g. Mechanical balances were used until 1984 but from 1985 Soehnle electronic digital scales were introduced.

Triceps skinfold thickness

Triceps skinfold was measured as recommended by Tanner and Whitehouse (1962), except that the midpoint between the tip of the acromion and olecranon was marked with the arm hanging straight instead of bent. From 1972 to 1978 two measurements were taken, but from 1979 onwards a single measurement was recorded.

Other measurements

These are described where necessary in this book, or methods can be found in the relevant publications from the study.

Questionnaire items

Validated questions were used when possible, for example the respiratory symptom questions in Chapters 6 and 10 which were adapted from those used in an earlier department study (Leeder *et al.* 1976). Father's social class was coded from standard questions about his current or last job and employment status, using the latest available Office of Population Censuses and Surveys' (OPCS) classification of occupations at each survey. With the exception of the food frequency questions from 1992 to 1994, which were in a self-coding form, the answers were coded within the department. Coding sheets were used from 1972 to 1976, following adverse publicity surrounding com-

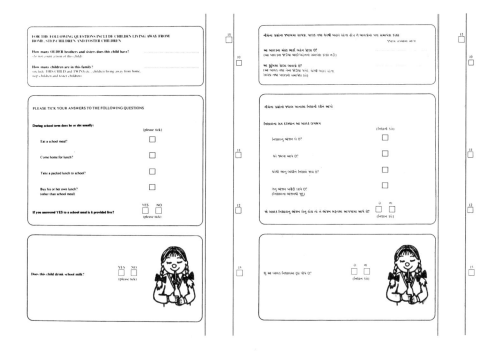

Fig. 2.2 Example of a page of the bilingual English/Gujarati questionnaire.

puterization of the UK 1971 census. From 1977 the coding boxes were on the questionnaire. Full pilot studies for the questionnaires were carried out in 1971 and 1976, prior to phase one and phase two, respectively.

Translations for inner-city areas and definition of ethnic group

Letters to parents were translated into all languages considered by the schools to be relevant, as described in Chapter 3. Questionnaires were translated into the main written languages, Urdu, Punjabi, and Gujarati for 1983 to 1991, with Bengali replacing Punjabi in 1993. The appropriate dual language questionnaire was sent to parents. As most answers required a box to be ticked or a number filled in relatively few questionnaire responses were sent for translation. An example page of the 1993 English/Gujarati new entrant questionnaire is shown in Fig. 2.2.

The corresponding section of the follow-up questionnaire was identical except for the omission of the question on the number of older brothers and sisters. The language spoken at home was recorded by the school and transferred to the data collection sheet used during fieldwork. Language spoken at home was used to define ethnic group as used in the NSHG. When the language was not an Indian subcontinent language the fieldworker's assessment was used to divide the children into white, Afro-Caribbean, or 'other'. Questions similar to those used in the 1991 census were included in the questionnaire for London areas at one survey of the inner-city sample, at the insistence of the Inner London Education Authority, but as questionnaires were not returned by the parents of all children who were measured this limited the usefulness of this information.

Quality control

Questionnaire

Except for the first 5 years, coding was carried out by the study fieldworkers—some of whom were also part of the analysis team, but all were full-time members of the study team. A system of check coding of 1 in 20 questionnaires was introduced to help maintain adherence to the coding constructions.

Measurements

Core measurements were taken by nurses employed locally in each area of the NSHG, supervised by a trained fieldworker. Quality control of measurements was achieved in two ways. A trial was held in a local primary school, which was not in the main study, to compare measurements taken by the fieldworkers on the same children prior to fieldwork. In most years three fieldworkers were employed, but occasionally a change of personnel during fieldwork was necessary. As well as supervising the measurements the fieldworker recorded a check measurement on 1 in 10 children. From 1973 to 1978 check measurements were taken alternately before and after the actual measurements for the selected children. In 1972 the check measurements were all taken after the actual measurements, and this was reintroduced in 1979 so as to maintain comparability of all the measurements used in analyses. The fieldworker trials, which are described below, consistently found a small bias towards height decreasing the more times a child was measured.

Results of the first two sets of check measurements were published (Irwig 1976), giving the distribution of absolute differences between measurements taken by nurses and fieldworkers. These were within ± 0.5 cm for height for over 95% of children, within ± 100 g for weight for over 90%, and within ± 1 mm for triceps skinfold for over 80%. The main value of the check measurements was to provide constant feedback to the nurses and fieldworkers on possible problems with measurement technique.

The most usual design for the annual fieldworkers' trial was for around 30 children to be measured three times, once consecutively by each of the fieldworkers, with the order of measurement randomized for children so that the six possible orders of measurement for the three fieldworkers were each allocated five times. When more than three fieldworkers were in the trial a balanced incomplete block design was used, so that no child had to be measured four or more times. The data were analysed within two working days, and when differences or large variations were apparent further training took place, and the trial repeated if necessary. The analysis of height by order of measurement showed differences, which were attributed to either the child or the stretcher relaxing slightly. The reduction from two to one triceps skinfold measurements was a consequence of a combination of the trial and check measurement results, which showed that two measurements taken by the same person showed little difference compared to two taken by different measurers, so that a second measurement by the same nurse added little. However, the trial data also showed that between-fieldworker variation was small in comparison to between-child variation; it is the latter which is relevant for analyses that utilize between-child variation. The intraclass correlation coefficient for triceps skinfold ranged from 0.95 to 0.99, over the trials from 1992 to 1994. In comparison, that for height was about 0.998 and for diastolic blood pressure it was 0.65. The Sub-committee on Nutritional Surveillance was not enthusiastic about triceps skinfold. Irwig (1976) seemed to think that the check measurement results showed considerable variation, and it became apparent that Department of Health officials thought it an unreliable measure. However the NSHG demonstrated that it was an extremely repeatable measure.

Measurements other than as described above were usually taken by the fieldworkers themselves, and assessed either in the regular trial or in a special pilot study.

Data management

Data were coded and transferred to punched cards from 1972 to 1981, or entered directly on to a computer file from 1982 onwards. Verification (double entry) was used throughout. All data were range checked, including by age for the measurements, edited, and rechecked. 'Impossible' measurements were set to missing, but other extreme values were retained unless found to be data entry errors. Cross-sectional, or 'flat' files were created for each year of survey, with dummy card images created when no questionnaire was returned or other records were missing. Sex and date of birth were usually recorded for children not measured because of parental refusal or persistent absenteeism; children who left the school prior to fieldwork were omitted when this was ascertained.

The authors of this book inherited a backlog of data cleaning, and the data for 1974 to 1976 were not linked to earlier years until after the 1977 fieldwork had started. Once discrepancies in sex and date of birth for children who were followed up had been resolved for these years, a system was introduced for linking each year to the previous year's data, checking for decreases in height and weight, as well as discrepancies in sex or date of birth. Those discrepancies that could not be resolved by the team were referred back to the school. Prior to the next survey, a list of children expected to be included—by name with survey number, sex, and date of birth—was supplied to the administrators within each area, to reduce the problem of wrong survey numbers. The most common problem encountered was for a child to be given its sibling's number instead of its own when its older sibling left the school.

A problem, common to all studies with a longitudinal component, was that as more follow-up data were added more errors were detected. With just two measurements of height it was not possible to determine which was in error if the second was less than the first measurement, but with some children having up to seven measurements during the period 1972 to 1982 it was often possible to determine which was out of step. An error in date of birth was sometimes undetected for more than one year. Every effort was made to correct records so that there was consistency throughout, but occasionally inconsistent information was obtained from the school, and even the sex remained undetermined for a few children whose names were unhelpful.

The number of records, of varying length, accumulated over the 23 years was 172 790. Most of the 87 424 eligible children had from one to three measurements, but a substantial number took part in five or six surveys in the first 10 years of the study.

As described earlier the follow-up questionnaire from 1984 onwards omitted questions in the full new entrant questionnaire that were independent of the child's age, such as birthweight and number of older siblings. These data were extracted from the file for the survey two years' earlier, the new entrant data being carried forward for a child for as many years as necessary.

Computing

In the early years there was no alternative to transferring the data to a remote mainframe at ULCC (University of London Computing Centre), and storing the data on magnetic tape. Incompatibility of tape format between the two ULCC machines at the time, the unreliability of tapes, and the subsequent changes of operating systems created difficulties that, thankfully, are completely outside the experience of computer users today. Data checking and editing were carried out via a suite of FORTRAN programs designed for the NSHG, which with modification stood the test of time until 1994. Gradually the introduction of mini-computers allowed the initial data checking to be carried out on machines locally, but the data files for each survey were assembled and analysed on remote faster machines with sufficient disk storage, the data being transferred from ULCC to the Manchester Computing Centre in the late 1980s.

Analysis was initially also carried out using locally written programs, but from 1977 GLIM and SAS were increasingly used, and more recently STATA, although some specially written software was required for the estimation of trends in growth.

Statistical analysis

As might be expected many of the analyses were cross-sectional multiple or logistic regression analyses of a single survey, or of the inner-city sample combined with an adjacent survey of the representative samples. Within such analyses the main statistical issue was how to express the outcome measure. Many of the analyses were of the measurements in relation to social factors, requiring inclusion of the whole sample for sufficient power to detect relatively small differences, but as height, weight, and triceps skinfold increase not only in mean value with age but also in variation, they should not be analysed by multiple linear regression without transformation.

Standard deviation scores

The expression of a child's height as SDS (standard deviation score), i.e. the difference between the measurement and an average value for the child's age and sex divided by the standard deviation appropriate for age and sex, was already common practice in 1972. Data were divided into 6-month age groups, and means and standard deviations of height within the groups were smoothed over age, for boys and girls separately. As height is Normally distributed at a given age for both adults and children, further transformation is not required.

Weight for a given age and sex is positively skewed. Rona and Altman (1977) used a shifted log transformation to normalize the distribution, with the constant dependent on age group and sex. Chinn and Morris (1980) modified this approach to construct weight SDS without discontinuities at age group boundaries. A weight-for-height SDS was then calculated as (weight SDS − b × height SDS)/RSD, where b was the sex-specific regression coefficient of weight SDS on height SDS, and RSD the sex-specific residual standard deviation.

Triceps skinfold SDS was calculated in a similar manner to that for weight for many of the early analyses, for example Morris and Chinn (1981) and Rona and Chinn (1982a).

Although description of the lung function measures obtained for 7–11-year-old children from 1987 to 1990 is postponed to Chapter 9, the statistical problems are explained here as their solution led to the development of a weight for height index. Lung function, as measured by FVC (forced vital capacity) and FEV_1 (forced expiratory volume in one second), increases with the height and age of children. The literature available in 1989 was inconsistent, some authors log transforming their data, and others stating that they needed no transformation as FVC and FEV_1 were Normally distributed for a given height. Multiple regression of each measure, whether log transformed or not, and whether height and age were also log transformed or not, fitted equally well. The publication of a paper by Bland et al. (1990) on birthweight and gestational age led to the realization that the problem was that FVC and FEV_1 had variance increasing with age or height, but were Normally distributed for given values of these. Hence the authors who worried about heteroscedasticity transformed their data and those who worried about Normality did not. Bland's solution for variables with these properties was to calculate expected values and residuals on the log scale, but to back-transform these before calculating SDS or centiles (Chinn and Rona 1992).

It was then realized that a similar approach could be used to calculate height SDS and reference curves (Chinn 1992), although a shifted log transformation was required to stabilize variance. This led to further consideration of weight and weight-for-height. The transformation log(weight – 9 kg) was found to stabilize variance over the age range 4 to 12 years (Chinn et al. 1992). The index $\log_{10}[(\text{weight} - 9)/\text{height}^{3.7}]$ was proposed as a measure of height, the coefficient of height in metres being derived from the optimal prediction of fatness as measured by triceps plus subscapular skinfold (Chinn et al. 1992). Age did not modify the index in any useful way. Over the age range 4 to 12 years the index has a number of advantages over BMI (body mass index), that is $\text{weight}/\text{height}^2$, as BMI in children is dependent on age and sex in mean value and variation (Cole et al. 1995), and hence unlike the weight-for-height index requires the calculation of smoothed means and variances by age. The mean of the index for English white boys and girls in 1990 was 0.831 and 0.841, respectively, with standard deviations of 0.066 and 0.079.

Calculation of triceps SDS in the later study years, and of normalized BMI when required, used the method of Cole (1988).

While adequate for cross-sectional analyses, the early calculations of weight and triceps SDS—and also those using the method of Cole (1988)—required several steps, and were specific to one survey. Parameters in the transformations were optimal for the year in question, but not for other surveys. Hence they were not ideal for the calculation of trends over time. The form of the outcome variable for the calculation of trends in height is described in Chapter 4, and those for weight, weight-for-height, and triceps skinfold in Chapter 5.

Calculation of trends using mixed longitudinal data

Measurements

The biggest statistical challenge was how to calculate trends over time in the core measurements, using all the data for the representative samples but taking into account the repeated measurements for the majority of the children. By about 1982, data had been assembled for the first nine years, and discrepancies found on longitudinal linking, as described above, had been removed as far as possible. This was before software became available for Generalized Estimating Equations (Zeger and Liang 1986), which allow a correlation structure to be specified for repeated measurements. Methods then available for longitudinal studies were not appropriate for an analysis of trends over time, which could have been estimated from a series of repeated independently sampled cross-sectional studies, with no longitudinal component. However, the distinction between longitudinal and cross-sectional objectives within one study was not well understood at the time, as discussed by Chinn (1989a).

For any one age group the calculation of a trend, say in height with time for 8-year-old children, was straightforward—as given that measurements were made a year apart, the number of children contributing more than one measurement was very small. By dividing children into year-of-birth cohorts, and defining nominal age as the year of measurement minus the year of birth, even the small number could be eliminated. Mean height for each cohort at each of the surveys where the cohort had a nominal age in the range 5 to 11 years was calculated, and a regression of mean height on time for each nominal age gave seven estimates of trend. These were then averaged to give an overall linear trend, and it was relatively straightforward to calculate the variances and covariances of the mean heights contributing to the final estimate, and hence a standard error for the estimate. Some refinements were made to allow for the mean age differing slightly from the nominal age as defined by the year of measurement and the year of birth. Details are given in the paper describing height trends from 1982 to 1990 (Chinn and Rona 1984), and a similar method was used for trends in weight, weight-for-height, and triceps skinfold (Chinn and Rona 1987a).

The same method was used in the final paper on trends in growth (Chinn et al. 1998a), as there seemed little to be gained by changing software at that point.

Respiratory symptoms

The problem of how to utilize all the respiratory symptom data to calculate trends in wheeze and attacks of asthma was similar except that the outcome was binary, not continuous. By the time this was tackled not only had a method been published (Woolson and Clarke 1984), but the software had been incorporated into SAS. Cohorts of children were defined by year of birth as in the analysis of trends in growth. The remaining details are described by Burney et al. (1990); the results are summarized in Chapter 11.

Changes in growth

Given the longitudinal component to the study, and the scarcity of such data when the NSHG began, it was natural that a number of analyses were carried out on changes in growth. When only one age group of children was included, as in investigating the influence of school milk on height gain (J. Cook et al. 1979), there was no problem in analysing height in one year with height the previous year as a covariate. However, when two or more age groups were combined the increasing variance of height meant that this straightforward analysis was not strictly valid. An analysis of change in SDS was used when investigating the relation of social factors to height gain (Smith et al. 1980), essentially showing whether or not social groups changed in relative position after 5 years of age or kept those established at an earlier age.

Efficiency of the design of the NSHG

When the inner-city sample was introduced in 1983 the consequent reduction in surveys of the representative samples from every year to every other year prompted calculation of the relative efficiency of the new design in relation to the original design (Chinn and Rona 1987b), and of mixed longitudinal designs compared to repeated independent cross-sectional studies (Chinn 1988). Particularly for height, but for all growth measurements, repeated measurements on the same child add less information than the same number of measurements on different children. The relative efficiency of different designs depends on the number of surveys, the number of age groups, how far apart the surveys are, the correlation between successive measurements on the same child, and the proportion of children followed-up. The method of analysis used for the trends in measurements over time enabled a calculation of the variance of the estimate with an assumption of the correlation for the individual measurements. For two measurements k years apart on the same child this was taken to be ρ^k, where a value of ρ of 0.99 is appropriate for height and 0.90 for weight. The loss of efficiency in changing from a one-year to a two-year cycle of surveys was found to be less than 50%, and in general the mixed longitudinal design was more efficient compared to independent cross-sectional surveys than might have been expected.

Effects of the cluster design of the NSHG

As described earlier in the chapter children were clustered within schools, which in turn were clustered within area or inner-city wards, although in most cases a single school represented the area or ward. While the effect of cluster sampling on a mean or prevalence estimate was well known in 1971 (for example Moser and Kalton 1971), no discussion of this has been found in the early documentation for the study, presumably because the main aim was to estimate trends over time rather than a population mean or prevalence.

The cluster design in relation to trends over time

The advantage of resurveying the same schools rather than resampling was that while the schools remained the same the primary question was whether to include area as a fixed effect in the analysis. Although, due to the computational difficulties this would have introduced at the time, area effects were not included, it is unlikely that results would have differed as cross-sectional analyses were unaffected (see below). The replacement of schools and areas was found to have little effect when trends were calculated with and without areas that were replaced, and most published estimates were based on all areas. Although variation in trends between areas within one sample was a possibility, this was less likely than differences in trends between social groups, which were represented in all areas.

The cluster design in relation to cross-sectional analyses

Almost all the cross-sectional analyses were at child level. There was lack of consistency in inclusion of area as a factor in the analyses, but, when studied, results were unaffected by inclusion of area as a fixed effect. Given the very large number of degrees of freedom in relation to those lost by treating area as a fixed effect rather than a random effect there would be little to gain by the latter approach. Very few analyses used variables at area level. Foster et al. (1983) related a child's height to population density based on ward data, and Chinn et al. (1989a) included latitude and longitude in an assessment of the need for new reference curves for growth. Certainly if the former analysis were now repeated multilevel modelling would be used (Rice and Leyland 1996), and it is unlikely that a relation between population density and a child's height would have been reported. Area variation in attained height is very small compared to other influences on a child's height, described in Chapter 6, or compared to unexplained variation, the intraclass correlation coefficient being of the order of 0.05.

The cluster design in relation to reference ranges

The NSHG data have been used to calculate reference ranges for growth, directly for the age range 5 to 11 years (Chinn and Morris 1980; Chinn et al. 1998b; Rona and Altman 1977), and in providing the bulk of that used in the calculation of UK standards (Cole et al. 1995; Freeman et al. 1995). Here it would have been appropriate to use weights calculated from the sampling probabilities, but as the schools were not chosen according to any random sampling scheme this was not possible. Chinn et al. (1998b) showed that for the haematological data collected for the 'rising-nine' children in 1994, the variation attributed to area was too small to have any effect of practical importance on reference ranges. As the previous UK growth standards were based on far fewer and less representative data (Tanner et al. 1966), no great concern was expressed over this point. In fact with an intraclass correlation of around 0.05 the area variation could have no appreciable effect on ranges for height.

Advantages and disadvantages of the chosen design

Clearly the design had its disadvantages. Had the schools been chosen randomly within employment exchange areas the NSHG could have been considered truly representative, with weighted estimates calculated when appropriate, and the design would not later have been criticized in the way it was towards its end. However, whether schools could have been chosen randomly is quite another matter, and whether co-operation would have been maintained yet another.

Random selection would have been essential had schools or areas been sampled each survey, i.e. if the study had been a series of independent cross-sectional cluster sample surveys rather than having the mixed longitudinal design. For the analysis of trends it would have been essential to regard area as a random effect, although otherwise the analysis would have been more straightforward. Random selection of individual children is preferable on grounds of statistical efficiency, as now used in the Health Survey for England (Prescott-Clarke and Primatesta 1997). However, lower response rates have been achieved in the Health Survey than in the NSHG, offsetting the nominal efficiency. Apart from little, if anything, being gained by resampling areas, a number of disadvantages of that design are evident. There would have been no longitudinal element to the data, which was exploited in several analyses, although not as originally envisaged by the Subcommittee on Nutritional Surveillance (Department of Health and Social Security 1973). This is discussed in Chapter 4. In addition, there would have been no shorter follow-up questionnaire to lighten the data collection load, the administrative effort would have increased and, perhaps of greatest importance, had the response rate decreased it would have been impossible to study whether this was uniform across all social groups.

Comparability of the data over time was of the first importance for a study designed to monitor trends in growth, and this was achieved through the high response rate for measurement and maintenance of the same schools and areas over long periods of time. Any disadvantages of the design seem to have been outweighed by the advantages, as concluded by Chinn (1995). Although with hindsight much that was done in the early years of the study might be carried out better, or differently, this is due largely to the enormous advances in technology, statistical methodology, software, and data management over the past 25 years.

3 The administration of long-term large studies

Requirements for long-term studies

The main aim of a long-term observational study, in which the same measurements are taken over time, is to be able to assess changes in the total group or within subgroups in a community. The requirements for fulfilling these objectives are that the measurements in the study are carefully described at the outset, that the same measurement techniques are maintained over time, that the fieldworkers are carefully trained in taking the measurements, and that the quality control of all procedures is assessed and maintained over time.

Appropriate measurements and questionnaires for achieving the aims of the study are very important, but are only part of the requirements. Good communication within the team, and with helpers in each NSHG study area in both schools and health authorities, is also very important. It is relatively easy to carry out a survey on a large group of individuals for one year or to follow a small number of children over a large period of time. It is more difficult to maintain continuous collaboration from a large number of schools and health authorities undergoing changes in structure and line of accountability, and amid changing health priorities and political support for the study. On top of all the requirements described above the information collected needs to be processed appropriately. Instructions for coding information should be unambiguous and clearly understood by the coders, and data have to be appropriately checked to ensure that information on children collected on more than one occasion are consistent.

Over the study period we complied with all the requirements enumerated above. Methods for conducting surveys have changed greatly over the last 25 years, but we feel that it may be helpful for prospective researchers to learn from the experience of the NSHG.

The team and the network of collaborators

The study team was small (Table 3.1). Over the last 18 years of the study there were three senior members of the department—a statistician, an administrator, and an epidemiologist—who were continuously involved with the study, but who also had other work commitments. Other personnel were part of the team for between 1 and 4 years, although one of the fieldworkers stayed with us for approximately 13 years. A second, more junior epidemiologist, was also a member of the team for approximately half of the study period.

Although the study team was small, the network of helpers in each study area was extensive. Contact with each study area was kept through our fieldworkers who each took responsibility for a third of the study areas. This ensured a prompt response to enquiries from helpers. We also gave the local collaborators in each of the participating areas the opportunity to discuss local and national results, and organizational issues, before starting an annual survey. The fieldworkers had an important role as ambassadors for the NSHG. They had ample opportunity for discussing issues that arose in the day-to-day running of the study. They contacted the most appropriate senior

Table 3.1   The study team

For the duration of the study
An epidemiologist
A medical statistician
A project administrator
Three fieldworkers
An assistant statistician
A secretary

For part of the study
A second epidemiologist
A fourth fieldworker
A second statistician

member of the team when an issue was not resolved satisfactorily. This level of autonomy gave job satisfaction to the fieldworkers during the period of preparation of the survey and during the data collection. The period of data coding was a less happy time. The task was seen as repetitive and unchallenging. This was the period of the year in which most of the conflicts and frustrations within the team came to the forefront. The excellent quality of the data available for analysis was due in great measure to the professional approach of most of the fieldworkers to both the interesting and the boring parts of the job and to the development of a good documentation system for all procedures in the study. A monthly administrative meeting during the periods in which fieldwork did not take place was helpful for discussing any issues relevant to the good functioning of the study.

The role of the administrator in large surveys which run for several years is very important. In the NSHG this person had to deal with a large number of invoices generated by the study preparation, expenses of members of the team visiting the areas, and expenses related to the activities of our helpers in every one of our 56 study areas. The administrator, who also performed a similar role for the whole department, had to respond to each of the requests for payment within a short time and at the same time exercise financial control over all expenses. To a large extent, the availability of such a person releases the researchers from administrative responsibilities so that they can focus on matters directly related to the scientific output of the study. In the NSHG an analysis meeting was held on a monthly basis. These meetings were attended only by those involved in the analysis of the data. The major purpose of these meetings was to monitor the progress of analyses and writing of papers as set against the current 2-year plan.

The headteachers and school nurses were essential for our maintaining contact with the areas before and after the period of data collection. Most of them were very supportive of the study. On the rare occasions when the headteachers or nurses did not want to continue the collaboration with the study we were able to hold further discussion, and on some occasions to reverse the decision to withdraw from the study through the good office of a specialist in public health medicine or a senior clinical officer. The excellent record of maintaining the same study areas (Table 2.1) was due to this extensive network of collaborators. The reasons for leaving the study were a school disappearing before or after redevelopment of the area, or lack of support from the headteacher or community health services. Support for the study from the headteacher was essential. Without it access to the school would have been very difficult. In some occasions, usually coinciding with a change of headteacher, there was unwillingness to collaborate because of concurrent administrative tasks related to the management of the school. In this situation the research team had to be prepared to facilitate tasks for the school. In Britain the school secretary is the key person in maintaining a link, and sometimes solutions to problems can be found through the goodwill of the school secretary.

Table 3.2   Annual ongoing activities

Preparation of questionnaires and forms
Manuals
    Administration manual including letters to parents
    Measurement manual
Preparation of selection of local and national results for each study area
Contact with each study area, and visit if necessary
Preparation of fieldwork activity
Training of fieldworkers in measurement techniques
Ensuring that all instruments were in working order
Preparation of the list of eligible children in each participating school
Distribution of questionnaires (up to three times)
Fieldwork
Data coding
Data entry
Data checks and resolution of inconsistencies
Data analysis and writing up reports and papers
Occasional activities
    Preparation of protocols
    Ethical approval from committees in each health district

Activities related to the study

Table 3.2 lists the activities related to the preparation of each survey as well as tasks during and after fieldwork. All the activities were carefully scheduled, as any delays in the preparation of the study had consequences for the success of the survey. The preparation cycle started in October each year, 7 months before the fieldwork started. Everybody in the team participated in the review of the questionnaire. Although we maintained the same core questions over the study period, we changed and added topics of interest in relation to child health. From 1977 onwards there was an emphasis on producing a fairly short questionnaire and only questions that had a clear purpose were included in the study. Changes to the questionnaire and measurements were discussed by all the team. In odd years when the inner-city areas were studied (see Chapter 2) the questionnaires were translated into the three minority languages that were most read in the study areas. These questionnaires were bilingual to facilitate completion. Thus parents could complete the questionnaire using the English or the translated version (Fig. 2.2). Very few parents used the translated versions of the question-naire, but we kept them to show our willingness to facilitate their response to the questionnaire. The letters explaining the study to parents were translated into 11 languages.

From November to February we reviewed all other explanatory material. There was an 'Administration manual', which provided information on the preparation of the fieldwork in relation to the distributions of the questionnaire, preparation of consent letters and forms to the parents, and information on the distribution of equipment for the measurement session. A 'Nurses manual' explaining each of the measurements in the study was also produced. The local nurses, many of whom participated in several surveys, took some of the measurements in the study. The fieldworker trained the local nurses in these measurements on the first morning of the survey.

An analysis was produced for each study area giving results comparing the children in their participating schools, or schools, with the study results as a whole. This was usually well received by the people in the study areas. As we offered to visit the study area in February or March our helpers received the material well before the following survey took place. At that visit we discussed issues related to the purpose and the administration of the study, and the most interesting national and local results.

From January to March the fieldworkers trained each other in the measurement techniques following the prepared protocols. One or two months before the start of a survey a trial was organized to ensure that agreement between fieldworkers in the measurement of height, weight, and triceps skinfold thickness was high (see Chapter 2). If agreement between fieldworkers was not satisfactory the cause of the disagreement was explored and remedial action decided. On a few occasions a second trial was carried out when the results of the first trial were unsatisfactory. We were usually satisfied that the fieldworkers' measurement techniques were similar by the time the survey took place. The fieldworkers were also responsible for checking all the equipment, to minimize the danger of malfunctioning equipment during fieldwork.

Fieldwork

Data collection took place each year from April to June and from September to November. The week of survey was agreed with each area at the time of recruitment, and almost without exception each subsequent survey in the area took place in the same week of the year. The questionnaires and letters were distributed approximately 3 weeks before the measurement sessions. The letters explained the reasons for the survey and asked parents to alert the school immediately if they did not want their child to be measured. A reminder was sent 2 weeks after the first distribution and, if necessary, a third distribution 3 weeks later. In some areas the third distribution was replaced by home visits. These were organized by local nurses and generally included about 3% of the children in each area. In a few inner-city areas with a high percentage of parents who had difficulties in completing the questionnaire a language liaison officer working with the school helped us to obtain a completed questionnaire from these parents. Home visiting was extensive in these areas.

The maximum time allocated to measurement sessions was 1 week in each study area. Longer periods would have had resource implications. The usual arrangement was that two local nurses, who were trained on the morning of the first day, took the measurements. The ability to take measurements between nurses was variable. However, most of them were proficient in taking all measurements as shown in the quality control system in the study. New measurements were included for studying risk factors for CHD (coronary heart disease) in 9-year-old children from 1992. These measurements were blood pressure, lipoprotein profile, cardiorespiratory fitness, and skinfold thickness at two other sites. From 1987 to 1990 we also included lung function measurements in 7–11-year-old children. These measurements were taken by the fieldworker. In 1994 we added red and white blood cell counts as well as haemoglobin and ferritin levels. Venepuncture was performed in separate sessions by a phlebotomist with experience in taking blood specimens from children.

There were some special features worthwhile mentioning in a multiethnic survey. Measurement of the height of children of Afro-Caribbean, Rastafarian, and Sikh descent is not straightforward. We needed to acquire special callipers to measure, and hence deduct, the extra height associated with plaits worn by Afro-Caribbeans, 'dread locks' worn by Rastafarians, and the 'patka' worn by older Sikh children (Rona 1995).

A list of children in each school was prepared locally, approximately 2 months before the start of fieldwork. To facilitate this, and to try to ensure that children retained their survey number, a list was supplied to each area of those children from the previous survey who were young enough to be still at primary school. Occasionally a child left the school before one survey, and returned by the following survey. One child even moved between schools in the NSHG, but into different study areas. The fact that these rare events were brought to our attention illustrates the dedication to the study of the local collaborators.

When the NSHG was enhanced in 1983 by a large sample of inner-city areas we asked the schools about the language spoken at home for each child. In some areas with a large percentage of children originating from the Asian subcontinent repeats of surnames, such as Patel and Singh, were a common finding. Unambiguous identification of children would have been very difficult without local help. At the end of the fieldwork in each area the fieldworker prepared a report highlighting problems and unusual events during the fieldwork.

Parental consent

When the NSHG started it was not routine to submit a community study to local ethics committees. In our study all parents were sent a letter. In this letter parents were advised that if they did not want their child measured they should inform the school immediately in writing ('immediately in writing' was in capitals and underlined). Parents could advise this verbally, but for record keeping we preferred a letter. Parents who made it clear that they did not want their child to participate in the study ever were kept on a separate list and were not invited to participate again. There were very few incidents or complaints in relation to the 87 424 children who were eligible to participate in the study at least once over the 23 years. The incidents were solved either by the fieldworkers themselves or by the headteacher—on very rare occasions, less than once a year, the co-ordinator or the study administrator was also involved. Complaints were always resolved within the network of the study.

The measurements related to coronary heart disease risk factors introduced in the 1990s required ethical approval (Chinn et al. 1998b; Hammond et al. 1994a). No ethics committee refused permission. Since we requested positive consent for these measurements the response rate was lower, approximately 75%. Parents were more reluctant to allow their children to provide a blood sample than to be measured. However, the rates in our study compare favourably to the rates of other studies in the UK (Prescott-Clarke and Primatesta 1997). We had no serious complaint related to these measurements. It is ironic that after obtaining ethical approval from all relevant ethical committees for piloting venepuncture and for the main survey, our first paper reporting results from the pilot study was rejected by the *Archives of Disease in Childhood* on the grounds that such a study was unethical. We challenged the basis on which such a decision was taken. It is to the credit of the journal that the editorial board not only reconsidered its decision, but published the paper followed by commentaries of paediatricians and researchers considering the ethics of venepuncture in healthy children from different perspectives (Hammond et al. 1994a and commentaries).

Communicating abnormal results to parents and doctors

Organizers of this type of study agonize over whether to contact parents, and over the threshold at which to contact parents, when a measurement is anomalous. All but one of the local ethics committees required such results to be reported; the remaining committee stipulated that parents should not be contacted, but the chairman changed his mind when contacted over the case of a child with a haemoglobin level of 9 g/dl. A paediatric endocrinologist approached us for information on a child's height for a period of five years. We provided the available information, and afterwards the doctor criticized us for not approaching health services and parents in cases when the child was too short for its age. We did so on a trial basis for a year. We found that parents were indifferent to the information provided and on a few occasions parents criticized us for approaching them about this issue, so we discontinued this service.

From 1992 we approached parents and their family doctors simultaneously when we detected a child whose blood pressure was too high, their red blood cell count too low, or their cholesterol level too high. On very few occasions we received an acknowledgement from the doctor. We were praised by a doctor for detecting a child with high blood pressure in whom a coarctation of the aorta was diagnosed, but in the large majority of cases we are unaware of the action taken as a result of our letter.

Parents' comments

The questionnaire to parents provided a box for comments, which was used for three main reasons: parents wanted to explain further an answer given in the questionnaire; they wanted advice in relation to a school or health issue; or they wanted to criticize the study. A common critical remark from parents was that they could not understand the reason why we asked so many questions on social background as they did not perceive any connection between their child's health and their socioeconomic position. On rare occasions parents criticized the Government for spending money on a survey when they perceived a lack of resources devoted to health and education. We waited to the end of the annual survey to reply to parents' comments. By the end of the study we were classifying comments into three groups, those that did not need a reply, those for which a standard letter was available (we developed a set of approximately 10 different standard letters), and a third group concerning an unusual issue.

Conclusions

Outside the research field, and sometimes within the field, it is not appreciated how much administrative preparation is required for a project to be successful. Concentration is on the aims of the project and the methodology. Unfortunately, projects based on good ideas and sound methodology, but where little attention has been paid to administrative details, are doomed. This is more so now that potential collaborators are under pressure to provide detailed information about the activities in which they are involved and are less willing to become involved in new long-term responsibilities. This chapter describes the steps we developed for making our study a success. Settings vary and requirements over time change. However, prospective researchers of large projects may learn from the experience of those who have been involved in previous studies.

4 Secular trend in height

Introduction

The NSHG was planned with the expectation that the height of the population would continue to increase naturally, and that failure to do so could be attributed to adverse economic circumstances. The Sub-committee on Nutritional Surveillance clearly envisaged that monitoring the rates of growth would be the primary outcome of the NSHG (Department of Health and Social Security 1973). The monitoring was expected to 'help to identify the effects of changes in food policy while any such effects are reversible'. The importance of monitoring individual children had been recognized for some time, and the increase in height had led to the updating of growth charts over a relatively short period of time (Tanner et al. 1966). The greater sensitivity of velocity over attained height for the detection of failure to thrive of the individual child had been recognized, no doubt influencing the Sub-committee's recommendation, although this has been challenged recently (Voss 1995). Extrapolation of what is best for the child to groups of children may be attributed to a failure to distinguish between population monitoring and the screening and surveillance of individuals, as the differences were not made explicit until much later (Goldstein and Tanner 1980).

However, it was realized by the study team in the early years of the NSHG that this was unrealistic for several reasons. First, there are analytical and interpretative difficulties in monitoring rates of growth rather than attained height (Chinn 1995). Rates of growth over successive time periods are negatively correlated, due to one measurement contributing to both variables. If a child leaving a school is immediately replaced by a child of the same age and gender entering the school no measurement of attained height is missing, but a contribution to the rate of growth is lost, so mobile children would be underrepresented. Of even more importance, it is not clear how a comparison of the mean growth rates of cohorts could be interpreted. Cohorts of children who start with the same mean height at 5 years of age, but who grow at different rates, will differ in attained height at a later age, and so a comparison of mean heights can provide the same information in a simpler form. On the other hand, if cohorts differ in mean height at 5 years of age then interpretation is difficult because it is known that, on average, taller children grow at a faster rate leading to the increasing between-child variation in height with age (Chinn 1992; Smith et al. 1980).

Second, there are limits on how far the height of an individual child can deviate from the norm, so a rather longer time period was required to detect changes in height than had been envisaged. Third, the effects of the changes in welfare policy that prompted the study were better addressed with analyses specifically designed for their estimation. In spite of these reservations, and with the proviso that attained height should replace rate of growth, the Sub-committee's conclusion that regular assessment would provide the most sensitive indicator available of nutritional status is not in dispute. The importance of height surveillance has been reflected in the number of papers from the NSHG that have wholly or in part reported on the secular trends in height.

Although the post-war population increases in height had been sufficient for clinicians to recognize, and had prompted the updating of growth standards (Tanner et al. 1966), there was a lack of comparable data in Britain that could be used to estimate precisely the changes in mean height, or to detect the size of the effect that might realistically be expected from changes in welfare provision. Except for school records, that were considered then (Holland, personal communication) and now (Voss 1995) to be inaccurate, nationally representative data were not available until the

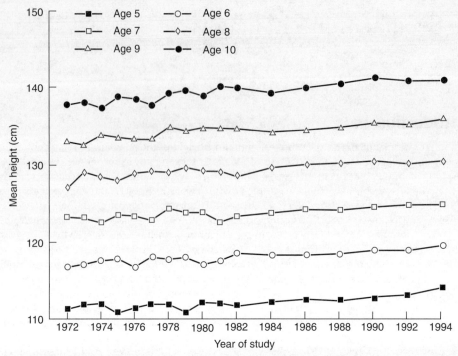

Fig. 4.1   Mean height of Scottish boys, 1972 to 1994. Taken from Hughes *et al.*, *Archives of Disease in Childhood*, 1997, **76**, 182–9; with permission from the *BMJ* Publishing Group.

establishment of the British birth cohort studies, and then only for limited ages. Tanner had used the London County Council 1959 survey of schoolchildren supplemented by a number of smaller studies to construct the growth standards. Although the 1946 and 1958 birth cohort studies each measured children at approximately 7 and 11 years of age, a comparison of mean height was not published until 1983 (Peckham *et al.* 1983). The enthusiasm at the time for longitudinal studies, both national and local (Tanner 1981), may have contributed to the choice of a mixed longitudinal design for the NSHG. National cross-sectional surveys had been conducted in a number of other countries prior to 1970 (Eveleth and Tanner 1976), but the NSHG was unique in contributing UK national data for a continuous age range.

Trends in the representative samples from 1972 to 1994

At the end of the study trends in height for the representative samples over the whole period were examined graphically. For this purpose the small numbers of non-white children were omitted, as were children younger than 5 years of age or those aged 11 years or over. Graphs of the mean height for each of the six age groups against the year of survey were given by Hughes *et al.* (1997), for boys and girls in England and Scotland. From 1983 onwards data for the 14 Scottish areas were combined and plotted as if all had been collected in the second, even, year. Figure 4.1 shows the results for Scottish boys. The smaller sample size in Scotland from 1972 to 1982 was responsible for the relative instability in the estimates for that period. As the size of the trend is small in relation to between-age variation in height, the small differences in trends between age groups are difficult to

Table 4.1 Mean height for English children in 1972 and 1994 (by age group), the difference, and 95% confidence interval (CI)

Age (years)	1972			1994		Difference in mean height (cm)	95% CI for difference (cm)
	n	Mean height (cm)		*n*	Mean height (cm)		
Boys							
5	564	111.95		462	112.83	0.89	0.27 to 1.50
6	609	118.20		442	119.04	0.84	0.20 to 1.48
7	649	123.79		494	124.92	1.14	0.50 to 1.77
8	617	129.40		461	130.70	1.30	0.59 to 2.01
9	607	133.64		387	136.88	3.24	2.45 to 4.04
10	593	139.84		402	141.32	1.48	0.67 to 2.30
Girls							
5	570	111.26		440	111.35	0.09	−0.54 to 0.72
6	585	117.12		442	118.41	1.29	0.64 to 1.95
7	624	122.79		453	124.39	1.60	0.92 to 2.28
8	571	128.33		403	129.69	1.36	0.58 to 2.13
9	537	133.86		374	135.61	1.74	0.89 to 2.60
10	576	139.57		434	141.36	1.79	0.93 to 2.65

Taken from Hughes *et al.*, *Archives of Disease in Childhood*, 1997, **76**, 182–9; with permission from the *BMJ Publishing Group*.

show graphically. The increasing trends were quite linear, but the lines for the six age groups were not totally parallel, in any of the four gender–country groups. This is clear in Tables 4.1 and 4.2 (reproduced from Hughes *et al.* 1997), which show the mean height for each age group in 1972 and 1994, the differences in means, and associated 95% confidence intervals. There was a greater increase in older children than in younger children, and a greater increase—of 2.67 cm (95% confidence interval 2.36 to 2.98 cm)—in Scottish children compared to English children where it was 1.39 cm (95% confidence interval 1.18 to 1.59 cm). Scottish children had been reported to be shorter than English children in 1972 (Rona and Altman 1977), but by 1990 the difference was minimal and not statistically significant (Chinn and Rona 1994).

Estimates of linear trend

The first estimates of linear trend in height from the NSHG were based on all available data from 1972 to 1980 (Chinn and Rona 1984), although a graphical analysis of data for three cohorts (Rona and Chinn 1982*b*) had already suggested that, in England at least, the secular trend was continuing. The 1984 paper developed and described the methodology for the estimation of trends from mixed longitudinal data, although some simplification was made in a subsequent paper (Chinn and Rona 1987*a*). It was concluded that a cubic polynomial could be use to describe changes in height with age, and the robustness of the estimates to the replacement of areas and schools taking part in the study was demonstrated. The estimates shown in the first column of Table 4.3 are taken from the 1987 paper using the simplified method, to be consistent with subsequent estimates, but differ little from those published in 1984. Boys showed a greater increase than girls over the early period of the

Table 4.2   Mean height for Scottish children in 1972 and 1994, by age group, the difference, and 95% confidence interval (CI)

Age (years)	1972		1994		Difference in mean height (cm)	95% CI for difference (cm)
	n	Mean height (cm)	n	Mean height (cm)		
Boys						
5	190	111.21	262	114.00	2.79	1.84 to 3.74
6	179	116.78	312	119.59	2.81	1.85 to 3.76
7	164	123.22	305	124.88	1.66	0.58 to 2.75
8	153	127.00	311	130.53	3.53	2.39 to 4.67
9	200	133.00	293	136.02	3.03	1.97 to 4.08
10	162	137.77	327	140.90	3.13	1.90 to 4.36
Girls						
5	165	111.11	289	113.02	1.91	0.98 to 2.85
6	152	115.58	286	118.26	2.69	1.65 to 3.73
7	170	122.00	315	124.08	2.09	1.05 to 3.12
8	164	127.47	293	129.96	2.49	1.37 to 3.60
9	155	132.34	288	135.58	3.24	2.07 to 4.41
10	172	137.99	314	140.72	2.73	1.49 to 3.98

Taken from Hughes *et al.*, *Archives of Disease in Childhood*, 1997, **76**, 182–9; with permission from the *BMJ* Publishing Group.

study, and Scottish boys a greater increase than English boys. Standard errors are shown rather than confidence intervals, so that all estimates can be shown in a single table, but 95% confidence intervals can be calculated as trend $\pm$ 2 standard errors.

The expectation at the outset that a cessation of the secular trend, or even a decrease in height, would be observed, was not realized. While there was continuing interest in whether the increase would be maintained there was also a desire to explain the increase. The method of analysis employed in the 1984 and 1987 papers was efficient in using all the mixed longitudinal data, but it did not lend itself to the inclusion of explanatory variables. A different approach was therefore adopted in the second analysis (Chinn *et al.* 1989*b*). So that the assumptions of independence for multiple regression analysis were met, three non-overlapping surveys were chosen: 1972, 1979, and 1986. The trends estimated for 1972 to 1979 and from 1979 to 1986 are shown in Table 4.3. They differ somewhat from the other estimates, which was subsequently ascribed to the fact that only data from schools participating throughout the period were included, thus increasing the sampling variation (Hughes *et al.* 1997). It is ironic that possibly the apparent cessation of trend from 1979 to 1986 was the only NSHG result to raise any real concern at the Department of Health. Price (1991) used the paper in a study of the dissemination and use of results from the NSHG. He quoted an interviewee at the Department of Health as saying that the paper was 'the most important ever produced by the NSHG', and described the view at the Department 'as one of mild concern tempered with caution'. He expressed the view (Price, personal communication) that without the cause for concern the Department of Health might have found reasons to stop the NSHG earlier.

A similar analysis for changes in weight-for-height and triceps skinfold thickness, but including all areas and schools, was carried out for 1972 to 1982, and for 1982 to 1990, which is described in

Table 4.3 Estimates (standard error) of annual linear secular trends in height (cm) for English and Scottish children

	1972–80[1] per cohort	1972–79[2] per year	1972–82[3] per year	1979–86[2] per year	1982–90[3] per year	1984–94[4] per cohort	1972–94[5] per year
English							
Boys	0.074 (0.018)	0.073 (0.022)	0.072* (0.017)	0.033 (0.024)	0.075* (0.021)	0.082 (0.016)	0.066 (0.007)
Girls	0.041 (0.019)	0.074 (0.024)	0.054* (0.017)	−0.017 (0.026)	0.113* (0.021)	0.088 (0.016)	0.055 (0.008)
Scottish							
Boys	0.137 (0.035)	0.159 (0.051)	0.144* (0.034)	0.017 (0.053)	0.157* (0.042)	0.136 (0.020)	0.126 (0.011)
Girls	0.045 (0.036)	0.134 (0.050)	0.102* (0.034)	−0.011 (0.054)	0.165* (0.042)	0.127 (0.021)	0.112 (0.011)

*Based on the assumption that one standard deviation score is approximately 6 cm.
[1]Chinn and Rona 1987a; [2]Chinn et al. 1989b; [3]Chinn and Rona 1994; [4]Chinn et al. 1998a; [5]Hughes et al. 1997.

Table 4.4   Estimates (standard error) of linear secular trends per annual cohort in height (cm) in English inner-city children 1983 to 1993

	Boys	Girls
White	0.123 (0.025)	0.163 (0.026)
Afro-Caribbean	0.152 (0.038)	0.115 (0.038)
Urdu/Punjabi	0.168 (0.030)	0.150 (0.031)
Gujarati	0.158 (0.056)	0.262 (0.061)
Other Indian	0.082 (0.069)	0.303 (0.074)

Taken from Chinn *et al.*, *Archives of Disease in Childhood*, 1998*a*, **78**, 513–17; with permission from the *BMJ* Publishing Group.

Chapter 5. For completeness, the report (Chinn and Rona 1994) included estimates of trends in height for these periods, from which two of the sets of estimates in Table 4.3 have been derived. The sixth set of estimates in Table 4.3 were calculated using all the mixed longitudinal data from 1984 to 1994 to compare with the trends for inner-city children (see below), and the final estimates were derived from just the 1972 and 1994 data (Hughes *et al.* 1997). The distinction between a per-cohort and a per-year estimate is derived from the method of estimation. As, once age changes are considered, linear period, and cohort effects are confounded the distinction is largely semantic.

With the exception of those from 1979 to 1986 the estimates are substantially in excess of twice their standard errors and broadly in agreement with each other, adding to the conclusion from the graphical analysis that the trend was reasonably linear over the whole time period. When explicit comparison was made between estimates based on data from schools continuing in the study and those replaced little difference was found (Chinn and Rona 1984, 1994), so those based on all schools are to be preferred. The time interval on which an estimate is based has the greatest influence on the precision of the estimate, with the use of all data rather than just two surveys reducing error by relatively little, due to the mixed longitudinal structure of the data and the very high correlation of height measured on two occasions for a child. However, in general, a trend based on several years' data is to be preferred to one based on just two surveys, either of which may be atypical by chance. If there was a real reduction in the trend between 1979 and 1986 it is clear that it was temporary, and that the increase in height of children aged 5–11 years continued up until 1994.

The NSHG is unable on its own to distinguish between an increase due to earlier maturation and an increase leading to greater adult height. The smaller increase for the youngest children (Chinn and Rona 1984) was first thought to indicate earlier maturation as the cause, but later evidence of an increase in adult height (Rona 1998) militated against this as the sole explanation.

Inner-city children 1983 to 1993

As the analyses of data from the representative sample had shown the need for several years' data to establish trends, these were not calculated for the inner-city sample until the end of the study. Even then standard errors were substantial for trends for Gujarati children. Height increased significantly for all groups of children except Other Indian boys (Table 4.4, taken from Chinn *et al.* 1998). The trends for the inner-city children were generally greater than those for the representative samples (Table 4.3, sixth column), and in particular for the ethnic minorities. Despite some catching up the Gujarati children remained the shortest at most ages. Ethnic group differences in attained height are discussed in Chapter 6.

Factors associated with trends

Changes in family structure, social class distribution, and mean birthweight and parental heights were considered as candidate factors for explaining the increases in height in the representative samples (Chinn *et al.* 1989*b*). Comparable data were obtained from the questionnaire self-administered by the parent or guardian at each survey. About 50% of the increase in height from 1972 to 1979 was accounted for by decreases in family size, with some contribution from increases in parental height and birthweight. A shift in social class towards non-manual occupations showed little association with the trends.

A separate question is whether there were different trends for different population groups, such as those defined by social class. Two analyses of data from selected cohorts (Rona and Chinn 1982*b*) or years (Rona and Chinn 1984*a*) concluded that there was little difference in trends between different social classes or for only children compared to those in large families, and that there was a slight narrowing of the gap between children of employed and unemployed fathers. Over the period of the study there was a considerable increase in unemployment reported by the parents, which in England was due to unemployment becoming more frequent outside the unskilled manual occupations (Rona and Chinn 1984*a*). The overall trend in height is composed of the trends in the separate groups compounded with a redistribution of the population over factors known to be associated with height differences.

There would appear to be a difference in trends either between white children and ethnic minority children, or between inner-city children and the representative population. As there were very few ethnic minority children included in the representative samples the two cannot be reliably distinguished, but the trend for white inner-city children is closer to that of the ethnic minority children than to that for white children in the representative sample. Coupled with the greatest trend being found for Gujarati girls it appears that trends are largest for the most deprived groups.

Conclusions

The NSHG provided the only real evidence of changes in the height of children in Britain over the period from 1972 to 1994. The initial expectation that a cessation of the secular trend might be observed was not realized, but there is no means of determining whether greater changes would have been observed under different economic circumstances. The power to detect differences in trends in the most deprived groups was low, leading to the recruitment of the inner-city sample in 1983. While there was evidence in favour of a narrowing of the gap between deprived and advantaged groups, whether defined by employment status or location of residence, this was small compared to the differences between groups in attained height.

Although there is an impression that studies on the secular trend of height in children are abundant, on close inspection most of the reports are based on cities, or combine information from surveys using different methodologies. In others, the data do not coincide with our period of surveillance or were not reported in mainstream scientific journals (Bodzsár and Susanne 1998). National data are available from the Czech Republic covering the period 1971 to 1991 (Vignerová and Bláha 1998). In the 5–9 year age range, height in most age groups increased approximately 0.1 cm per year from 1971 to 1991, slightly higher than in the English representative sample, and similar to the Scottish representative sample, but lower than in our inner-city sample. Socioeconomic circumstances over the period under consideration were very different in Britain and the Czech Republic. Although a single-centre study in the USA, the Bogalusa heart study provides data based on a society with a high standard of living. The height of 5–9-year-old children increased by 0.053 cm per year from 1973 to 1994 (Freedman *et al.* 1997), but this was averaged over boys and girls, and white and black children. There were greater increases in black children than in white, but figures are given only for the entire age range from 5 to 24 years. The CDC (Centers for Disease Control) Pediatric Nutrition Survey of low-income children from 1980 to 1989 (Yip *et al.* 1993) showed stable height for black and white children aged 2–5 years and an increase for Asian refugee children. However, one figure shows the latter group reaching the level of the white children by 1989 and another shows differences between the ethnic groups in 1989 across the same age range, so although this may provide evidence of a greater increase in a deprived group the results are uncertain.

While trends in Britain may be greater than in the United States it is certain that attained height is still less. White and black girls aged 9 and 10 years measured in Cincinnati and Berkeley prior to 1994 (Campaigne *et al.* 1994) were taller than NSHG children in 1994. It may be the case that children in Britain are close to reaching their growth potential. However, there is no evidence for a cessation of the trends in Britain. The Health Survey for England (Prescott-Clarke and Primatesta 1997) should allow future trends for English children to be estimated, and a comparison of the NSHG 1994 data with that of the 1995–1997 Health Survey has been carried out (Bost *et al.*, 1998). However, as the sampling strategy differed from that of the NSHG it would be unsafe to calculate trends spanning the two studies, and given the size of the trends (Table 4.3) several years' data from the health survey will be required before any difference from these can be detected. The health survey for England was designed to be nationally representative, whereas the prime aim in the NSHG was to collect comparable data over time. However, the Health Survey for England will provide little information on ethnic minority children. Information on the catch-up growth of ethnic minority and deprived groups in Britain is unlikely to be available in the near future.

5 Secular trend in obesity

Background

Although the Subcommittee on Nutritional Surveillance emphasized the monitoring of linear growth, annual measurement of weight and triceps skinfold thickness was incorporated into the initial protocol (Department of Health and Social Security 1973). As with height, monitoring of rates of change was envisaged, but it was recognized that weight gain could be transient in individuals, and that 'an acceleration in the rate of gain in weight can be a sign of increasing obesity, and not of improved health'.

Department of Public Health Medicine internal documents show that, at first, the study team's concern was with undernutrition as a result of changes in welfare policy, but this soon changed to an emphasis on the detection of increasing obesity. Unlike height, weight is relatively easy to measure accurately, but trends in weight cannot be interpreted without concurrent data on height. Data for weight-for-height were available at the inception of the NSHG but only from the same limited sources as described for height, and data on skinfolds were even more scarce. Triceps skinfold thickness requires careful training of fieldworkers, but in skilled hands is a more reliable measure than commonly thought. The Bogalusa heart study (Foster et al. 1980) reported a within-observer intraclass correlation coefficient of 0.97. Similar excellent repeatability in the NSHG led to a reduction in the number of measurements taken from two to one in 1979, as described in Chapter 2.

Although decisions were required for the analysis of trends in height in relation to the mixed longitudinal structure of the data, and over the construction of standard deviation scores to allow for the increasing variation of height with age, these were minor compared to those required for the analysis of weight-for-height and triceps skinfold. There was no consensus on how to adjust weight-for-height in children, a subject still controversial, nor any agreement on a cut-off point to define an obese child. Inevitably, therefore, different analytical approaches were adopted in the NSHG at different times, and methodology evolved. However, the main conclusions were undoubtedly independent of this. We were consistent in not using body mass index (BMI), which not only changes in mean value with age in children, but in variation and skewness (Cole et al. 1995).

Trends in representative samples from 1972 to 1994

Trends in weight, weight-for-height, and triceps skinfold thickness were published in graphical form alongside those for height (Hughes et al. 1997). Weight increased for English and Scottish boys and girls, but showed some variation with age group, broadly in line with the trends for height. However, as weight differences cannot be interpreted except in relation to height, further details are not given here. Weight-for-height was analysed using the index $\log_{10}[(\text{weight} - 9)/\text{height}^{3.7}]$, where weight is measured in kilograms and height in metres (Chinn et al. 1992). Details were given in Chapter 2. The index was designed to be independent of age, but this did not preclude trends that differed between age groups. Mean values were plotted for three 2-year age groups (Hughes et al. 1997), as shown for English boys in Fig. 5.1. The youngest English boys showed a slight decrease, the middle age group stayed stable, and the oldest showed an increase. English girls also showed trends increasing with age group, but with the youngest relatively stable and a small increase in the

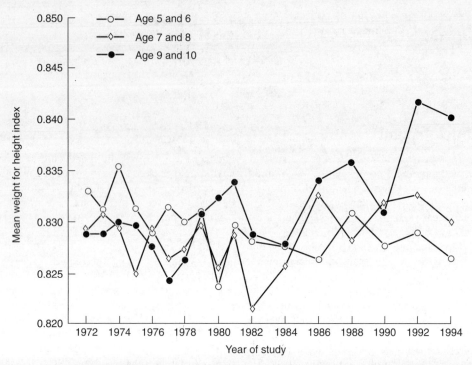

Fig. 5.1   Mean weight-for-height index of English boys, 1972 to 1994. See text for the definition of the index. Taken from Hughes *et al.*, *Archives of Disease in Childhood*, 1997, **76**, 182–9; with permission from the *BMJ* Publishing Group.

7- and 8-year-olds. Scottish children showed greater increases than English children, again girls more than boys. Tables 5.1 and 5.2 give the means for 1972 and 1994, from which it can also be seen that in 1972 Scottish children were lighter for their height than English children, but by 1994 the positions had reversed.

Triceps skinfold thickness showed a clear upward trend in almost all age groups for English and Scottish children (Tables 5.3 and 5.4). Figure 5.2 shows the trends for English boys, which is in marked contrast to those shown in Fig. 5.1 for weight-for-height. There were some notable differences from the trends in weight-for-height for all four gender–country groups. Trends in all age groups were positive, and more of the changes from 1972 to 1994 were statistically significant than for weight-for-height. English girls showed a smaller increase than English boys. Increases were greater in Scotland than in England, but the trends were not linear; for both Scottish boys and girls there was a plateau from 1986 onwards. The increases for Scottish girls, of more than 10% for each age group, were greater than those for Scottish boys except in one age group. The apparent temporary increase in the measurements for the youngest children in 1977 and 1978 seen in the figure was unexplained.

Estimates of linear trend

The first estimates of linear trends in weight-for-height (Chinn and Rona 1987*a*), for the period 1972 to 1980, were published well before the development of the weight-for-height index (Chinn

Table 5.1 Mean weight-for-height index for English children in 1972 and 1994, by age group, difference, and 95% confidence interval (CI)

Age (years)	1972			1994		Difference in mean weight-for-height	95% CI for difference
	n	Mean weight-for-height		n	Mean weight-for-height		
Boys							
5	563	0.834		460	0.826	−0.007	−0.02 to 0.00
6	607	0.833		442	0.827	−0.006	−0.01 to 0.00
7	648	0.830		491	0.829	−0.001	−0.01 to 0.01
8	614	0.828		461	0.831	0.002	−0.01 to 0.01
9	604	0.827		387	0.836	0.009	−0.00 to 0.02
10	593	0.830		402	0.844	0.014	0.00 to 0.02
Girls							
5	570	0.823		440	0.827	0.004	−0.00 to 0.01
6	583	0.833		441	0.828	−0.005	−0.01 to 0.00
7	622	0.832		451	0.838	0.006	−0.00 to 0.01
8	571	0.832		402	0.837	0.005	−0.01 to 0.02
9	537	0.840		371	0.854	0.014	0.00 to 0.02
10	576	0.840		432	0.852	0.012	0.00 to 0.02

Taken from Hughes *et al.*, *Archives of Disease in Childhood*, 1997, **76**, 182–9; with permission from the *BMJ* Publishing Group.

Table 5.2 Mean weight-for-height index for Scottish children in 1972 and 1994, by age group, difference, and 95% confidence interval (CI)

Age (years)	1972			1994		Difference in mean weight-for-height	95% CI for difference
	n	Mean weight-for-height		n	Mean weight-for-height		
Boys							
5	188	0.831		260	0.833	0.002	−0.01 to 0.02
6	179	0.825		311	0.827	0.002	−0.01 to 0.01
7	162	0.826		305	0.831	0.004	−0.01 to 0.02
8	152	0.832		310	0.838	0.006	−0.01 to 0.02
9	199	0.828		292	0.847	0.019	0.01 to 0.03
10	161	0.823		326	0.842	0.019	0.01 to 0.03
Girls							
5	164	0.816		289	0.826	0.010	−0.00 to 0.02
6	151	0.816		286	0.832	0.016	0.00 to 0.03
7	167	0.815		315	0.837	0.022	0.01 to 0.04
8	164	0.827		292	0.852	0.025	0.01 to 0.04
9	155	0.831		288	0.856	0.025	0.01 to 0.04
10	172	0.836		313	0.865	0.028	0.01 to 0.04

Taken from Hughes *et al.*, *Archives of Disease in Childhood*, 1997, **76**, 182–9; with permission from the *BMJ* Publishing Group.

Table 5.3 Geometric mean triceps skinfold thickness (GM) for English children in 1972 and 1994, by age group, the percentage change, and 95% confidence interval (CI)

Age (years)	1972		1994		% Change	95% CI for % change
	n	GM (mm)	n	GM (mm)		
Boys						
5	567	8.60	459	8.91	3.60	0.48 to 6.83
6	610	8.30	439	8.69	4.69	1.51 to 7.96
7	648	8.23	493	8.88	7.92	4.33 to 11.64
8	616	8.39	461	9.05	7.93	4.00 to 12.01
9	608	8.82	387	10.29	16.60	11.46 to 21.99
10	592	9.30	405	10.86	16.71	10.81 to 22.92
Girls						
5	570	10.27	442	10.58	3.07	−0.03 to 6.27
6	585	10.35	439	10.63	2.67	−0.82 to 6.29
7	622	10.69	452	11.45	7.13	3.35 to 11.05
8	571	11.40	402	11.68	2.53	−1.74 to 6.99
9	536	12.12	372	12.96	6.89	2.22 to 11.78
10	575	12.93	431	13.73	6.26	1.63 to 11.09

Taken from Hughes *et al.*, *Archives of Disease in Childhood*, 1997, **76**, 182–9; with permission from the *BMJ Publishing Group*.

Table 5.4 Geometric mean triceps skinfold thickness (GM) for Scottish children in 1972 and 1994, by age group, the percentage change, and 95% confidence interval (CI)

Age (years)	1972		1994		% Change	95% CI for % change
	n	GM (mm)	n	GM (mm)		
Boys						
5	190	8.56	259	8.98	4.96	0.77 to 9.32
6	179	7.98	312	8.66	8.47	4.09 to 13.02
7	163	8.11	304	8.90	9.72	4.46 to 15.25
8	153	8.35	313	9.45	13.16	6.77 to 19.93
9	200	8.44	293	10.45	23.81	16.87 to 31.16
10	161	9.12	328	10.60	16.25	9.52 to 23.39
Girls						
5	164	9.38	281	10.67	13.80	9.04 to 18.77
6	152	9.29	282	10.42	12.22	7.33 to 17.34
7	170	9.97	313	11.13	11.63	5.79 to 17.80
8	164	10.46	291	12.36	18.18	11.23 to 25.77
9	155	11.18	289	13.32	19.09	11.86 to 26.79
10	172	11.75	314	14.31	21.76	14.56 to 29.42

Taken from Hughes *et al.*, *Archives of Disease in Childhood*, 1997, **76**, 182–9; with permission from the *BMJ Publishing Group*.

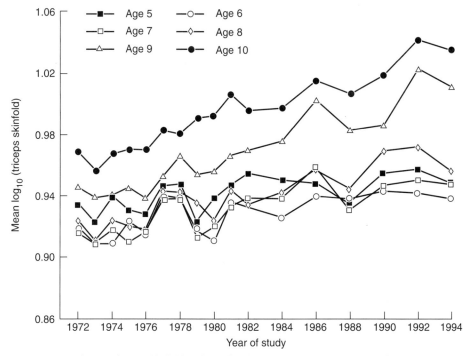

Fig. 5.2 Mean $\log_{10}$(triceps skinfold) of English boys, 1972 to 1994. Taken from Hughes *et al.*, *Archives of Disease in Childhood*, 1997, **76,** 182–9; with permission from the *BMJ* Publishing Group.

et al. 1992). The small increases in weight reported for English children up to 1982 were less than expected for their increases in height, as shown by the decreases in weight adjusted for height in the first column of Table 5.5, and the decreases in the weight-for-height index in column two. Scottish children, or at least the girls, tended to gain weight by more than was expected from their increase in height. From 1982 onwards all four groups increased in weight by more than was expected for their height, especially girls in both countries. Since the trends were not linear over the whole period (Chinn and Rona 1994) no overall estimate is given.

Estimates of the percentage increase per cohort in triceps skinfold thickness for 1972 to 1980 and 1984 to 1994 are given in Table 5.6. Chinn and Rona (1994) published trends in SDS from 1972 to 1982, and from 1982 to 1990, but these cannot be simply converted to percentage increases. The estimates confirm the conclusions drawn from the graphs that fatness, as measured by triceps skinfold thickness, stabilized over the latter period of the study in Scottish children, and that the trend may have been diminishing in English girls. English boys, however, appeared to still be increasing in obesity until 1994.

Inner-city children 1983 to 1993

All inner-city children increased in weight from 1983 to 1993 by more than expected for their height increase (Table 5.7) except for white boys, although only white and Gujarati girls showed a significant increase in weight-for-height. White inner-city children showed a decrease in triceps skinfold thickness, while all three groups of girls of Indian subcontinent origin increased

Table 5.5 Estimates (95% confidence interval) of annual linear secular trends in weight-for-height for English and Scottish children

	1972–80[1]	1972–82[2]	1982–90[2]	1984–94[3]
		Weight-for-height index ($\times 10^{-3}$)		
	% per cohort	per year	per year	per cohort
English				
Boys	−0.08 (−0.19 to 0.03)	−0.40 (−0.68 to −0.12)	0.50 (0.14 to 0.86)	0.54 (0.18 to 0.90)
Girls	−0.04 (−0.15 to 0.06)	−0.20 (−0.48 to 0.08)	1.13 (0.77 to 1.49)	1.02 (0.60 to 1.44)
Scottish				
Boys	0.11 (−0.09 to 0.32)	−0.20 (−0.92 to 0.52)	1.88 (1.04 to 2.72)	0.46 (0.02 to 0.90)
Girls	0.12 (−0.08 to 0.33)	1.00 (0.16 to 1.84)	1.63 (0.79 to 2.47)	1.15 (0.63 to 1.67)

[1]Chinn and Rona 1987*a*; [2]Chinn and Rona 1994; [3]Chinn *et al.* 1998*a*.

Table 5.6 Estimates (95% confidence interval) of annual linear secular trend in triceps skinfold thickness for English and Scottish children

	1972–80[1] (% per annual cohort)	1984–94[2] (% per annual cohort)
English		
Boys	0.44 (0.26 to 0.62)	0.44 (0.27 to 0.62)
Girls	0.21 (0.03 to 0.39)	0.12 (0.05 to 0.45)
Scottish		
Boys	0.85 (0.54 to 1.17)	0.01 (−0.20 to 0.22)
Girls	0.94 (0.59 to 1.29)	−0.14 (−0.34 to 0.06)

[1]Chinn and Rona 1987*a*; [2]Chinn *et al.* 1998*a*.

Table 5.7 Estimates (95% confidence interval) of linear secular trend per annual cohort in the weight-for-height index ($\times 10^{-3}$) in inner-city children from 1983 to 1993

	Boys	Girls
White	−0.26 (−0.82 to 0.30)	1.07 (0.37 to 1.77)
Afro-Caribbean	0.02 (−0.94 to 0.98)	0.11 (−1.05 to 1.27)
Urdu/Punjabi	0.59 (−0.33 to 1.51)	0.87 (−0.05 to 1.79)
Gujarati	1.01 (−0.59 to 2.61)	1.85 (0.03 to 3.67)
Other Indian	1.10 (−0.84 to 3.04)	1.88 (−0.28 to 4.04)

Taken from Chinn *et al.*, *Archives of Disease in Childhood*, 1998*a*, **78**, 513–17; with permission from the *BMJ* Publishing Group.

Table 5.8 Estimates (95% confidence interval) of linear secular trend in triceps skinfold thickness in inner-city children from 1983 to 1993

	Boys (% per annual cohort)	Girls
White	−0.48 (−0.74 to −0.23)	−0.45 (−0.72 to −0.18)
Afro-Caribbean	0.05 (−0.42 to 0.52)	0.20 (−0.27 to 0.29)
Urdu/Punjabi	0.07 (−0.30 to 0.45)	0.41 (0.08 to 0.74)
Gujarati	0.45 (−0.23 to 1.13)	1.12 (0.50 to 1.74)
Other Indian	−0.01 (−0.80 to 0.78)	0.84 (0.02 to 1.63)

Taken from Chinn *et al.*, *Archives of Disease in Childhood*, 1998*a*, **78**, 513–17; with permission from the *BMJ* Publishing Group.

significantly (Table 5.8). Weight-for-height does not only reflect fatness, as discussed in Chapter 7, so the differences in trends shown by weight-for-height and triceps skinfold thickness are not in conflict. Confidence intervals for the inner-city groups were wide, and estimates not statistically significant do not exclude increasing obesity.

Factors associated with trends

As with height the increasing trend in triceps skinfold was first observed graphically (Rona and Chinn 1982*b*, 1984*a*), but increases in weight-for-height were not detected in these analyses. No differences in the trends between social groups were observed. In an analysis similar to that carried out for height (Chinn *et al.* 1989*b*) several factors were considered as candidates to explain the trends in weight-for-height and triceps skinfold thickness, using data from 1972, 1982, and 1990 (Chinn and Rona 1994). As well as birthweight, family size and social class, parental BMIs, child in a one-parent family, mother's age at child's birth, and mother's education were included as potential explanatory variables. Trends in parental BMIs and decreasing family size were associated with up to a third of the increase in weight-for-height and triceps skinfold from 1972 to 1990 in Scottish children, but little of the trends for English girls, or in triceps skinfold for English boys, could be explained. Some differences in trends were found between social groups, but these were not consistent.

The factors associated with different trends in obesity are, first, the country of residence—in that children living in Scotland have shown greater trends in weight-for-height than children living in England, but who appear to have stopped increasing in fatness as assessed by triceps skinfold thickness. Second is ethnic origin—children of Indian subcontinent origin show greater increases in weight-for-height than either white or Afro-Caribbean children living in inner-city areas. Third, gender—girls of Indian subcontinent origin have greater increases than boys in triceps skinfold thickness.

Conclusions

It was not surprising that the NSHG soon identified increasing obesity, rather than undernutrition, as a major problem, as an increase in weight-for-height was found on comparing 7- and 11-year-old children between the 1946 and 1958 birth cohorts (Peckham *et al.* 1983). The conclusion (Hughes *et al.* 1997) that triceps skinfold is a more sensitive indicator of obesity than weight-for-height is extremely important, given the reliance on BMI in the Health Survey for England (Prescott-Clarke and Primatesta 1997). The reasons for the insensitivity of weight-for-height, and the ethnic group differences in the two measures, are discussed in Chapter 7.

Although no continuous monitoring system exists in the United States, four national surveys provide evidence of an increase in weight-for-height in black and white children aged 6–11 years from 1963 to 1991 (Troiano *et al.* 1995). Centiles of BMI defined by the earliest study were used, despite criticism by the authors of the use of BMI for children or adolescents. An earlier study of the first three of the four surveys (Gortmaker *et al.* 1987) used centiles of triceps skinfold to show an increase in obesity in 6–11- and in 12–17-year-olds. A separate research group (Harlan *et al.* 1988) found no corresponding increase in weight-for-height in the 12–17-year-olds, and attributed this to problems in the measurement of triceps skinfold thickness. As Troiano *et al.* (1995) found an increase in weight-for-height in this age group as well as in the younger children, and no conflict necessarily exists, there seems little doubt that obesity, however defined, has continued to increase in the United States, both for black and white children. This highlights the problem of relying on just one of these two complementary measures, and particularly on weight-for-height, and also on the dangers of drawing conclusions from a limited number of surveys. By plotting median triceps skinfold, Eveleth and Tanner (1990) concluded that there had been no increase between the first two National Health and Nutrition Examination Surveys (NHANES I and II).

Our results of no significant increase in weight-for-height or triceps skinfold in Afro-Caribbean children are not in line with the trends for black children in the United States, and are one welcome message from the NSHG. However, the confidence intervals are wide, and do not preclude increases as great as those seen in the representative white sample. In contrast, the increases seen in Indian subcontinent girls are worrying given the high mortality rates for coronary heart disease in that group in Britain (Balarajan 1991). Although the increases may represent catch-up growth, the mean weight-for-height index and mean triceps SDS are still below those of the other groups (Chinn *et al.* 1998*a*).

As for height, the Health Survey for England should eventually establish trends for weight-for-height, but not separately for ethnic minority groups; triceps skinfold was not measured. As was discussed in Chapter 4 there were differences in sampling between the health survey and the NSHG. In addition, in the health survey children were measured after removing shoes, heavy outer garments such as jackets and cardigans, heavy jewellery, loose change, and keys (Prescott-Clarke and Primatesta 1997), but not other clothing; in the NSHG children were measured wearing only underpants. For the comparison of the NSHG with the Health Survey an adjustment for clothing has been made (Bost *et al.*, 1998).

Our results have given warning that targets for a reduction in obesity are unlikely to be met (Hughes *et al.* 1997) and have shown the need for continued monitoring, especially of ethnic minority groups. However, trends in obesity are not confined to particular social groups, and prevention programmes should be aimed at the whole population.

6 Factors related to height

Background

Height was the most important measurement in the NSHG. The first report by the Sub-committee on Nutritional Surveillance (Department of Health and Social Security 1973) proposed a study of linear growth as the first objective, and the use of changes in weight as ancillary information. The Sub-committee's main concern was related to undernutrition. The second report of the Sub-committee (Department of Health and Social Security 1981) reiterated this by stating that even small changes in height may have important long-term consequences. Hence one of the main objectives of the NSHG at its outset was to assess the factors that influenced height and height gain, in particular the contribution of socioeconomic factors to the variation of height in Britain. However, variables such as parental heights, child's birthweight, and maternal age at the child's delivery, which reflect the effect of genes and the uterine environment on height, were also included in the analysis (Rona 1981). In practice, it is not clear whether any variable in this context is solely representing either the environment or genes (Rona and Chinn 1995). Thus the association between a child's and their parents' height may not only reflect a genetic association, but also an environment shared by the two generations.

Over the 23 years of the study a large number of papers were published on factors associated with height. The findings can be classified into four groups:

(1) ethnic group differences;

(2) factors associated with height without a specific hypothesis;

(3) the study of the association of a particular social factor and height;

(4) the study of the association of childhood illness or health-related behaviours and height.

Ethnic group differences are reported first, as, although these were not studied until the inner-city sample was introduced in 1983, ethnic group is one of the factors most strongly associated with height, and social factors within the inner-city sample cannot be described without taking account of ethnicity.

In most of the studies attained height was the independent factor in the analysis. However, we assessed height gain in relation to social factors, school milk and school meals, and childhood illness. Results in relation to school meals and school milk are reported separately in Chapter 13, those in relation to parental smoking are discussed in Chapter 10, and the relation of a child's height to the parental perception of food intolerance in Chapter 12. In all analyses of children's height reported in this chapter we used SDS to adjust for gender and increasing mean and standard deviation of height with age in the analyses, as described in Chapter 2. One SDS is equivalent to 5 cm in 5-year-olds and approximately 7 cm in 11-year-old children.

Ethnic group differences

We were the first to demonstrate large differences between ethnic groups in Britain, in the analysis of the 1982 and 1983 data (Rona and Chinn 1986). Figure 6.1 is based on data from the last two

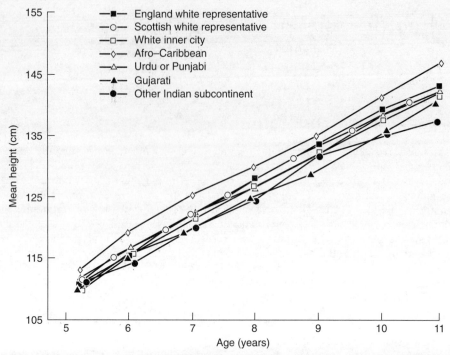

Fig. 6.1 Mean height plotted against mean age for boys in the 1993–94 surveys. Taken from Chinn *et al.*, 1998*a*, *Archives of Disease in Childhood*, **78**, 513–17; with permission from the *BMJ* Publishing Group.

years, 1993 and 1994. Despite a slight catch-up in height of those ethnic groups with the lowest average height in 1983 the differences in height have remained. Afro-Caribbean children were taller than children from any ethnic group. Their mean height was consistently above the 50th centile of the representative sample. We were also able to show that children from the Gujarati and Other Indian groups were the shortest among the ethnic groups studied. The mean heights of these children were between the 10th and 50th centile of the NSHG reference group. The white children as well as the Punjabi and the Urdu groups of the inner-city sample were of similar height, but slightly below the English and Scottish representative samples.

General overviews of factors associated with height

The major findings of factors associated with height were reported in three papers (Gulliford *et al.* 1991; Rona and Chinn 1986; Rona *et al.* 1978). Rona *et al.* (1978) described the variables related to height in 1972 in Scotland and England. Rona and Chinn (1986) studied the factors associated with height in the inner-city areas in 1983, and Gulliford *et al.* (1991) studied the variables associated with height in the three samples using the 1987 and 1988 data. The findings in the three studies were consistent in relation to the main factors associated with height. The most recent results (Gulliford *et al.* 1991) are reported here, with additional information on details that differed, or were not described in the 1991 analysis, from the other publications. The earlier analyses considered fixed sets of variables, with alternative models in the second report (Rona and Chinn 1986), while

Table 6.1 The impact of the principal factors associated with child's height

Variable	Representative samples	Inner-city sample
	Estimate from multiple regression (SDS)	
Maternal height (10 cm difference)	0.48	0.39
Paternal height (10 cm difference)	0.41	0.31
Birthweight (1 kg difference)	0.33	0.36
Length of pregnancy (compared to ⩽ 37weeks)		
38–42 weeks	−0.15	−0.19
>42 weeks	−0.50	−0.28
Family size (compared to 1 child)		
2	−0.14	Interaction
3	−0.22	with ethnic
4	−0.29	group
⩾ 5	−0.34	
Maternal age at delivery (compared to mothers ⩽ 19 years)		
20–23 years	−0.01	0.03
24–27 years	0.01	0.06
28–31 years	0.06	0.16
⩾ 32 years	0.12	0.28
School meals (compared to free school meals)		
Paid for	N/A	0.13
No school meal	N/A	0.06
Maternal employment (compared to employed mother)		
Housewife	−0.14	N/A
Not employed	−0.19	N/A

1.0 SDS is approximately 5–7 cm in the age range 5 to 11 years.
N/A stepwise multiple regression eliminated this variable.
Adapted from Gulliford et al., Archives of Disease in Childhood, 1991, **66**, 234–40; with permission from the BMJ Publishing Group.

Gulliford et al. (1991) started with a comprehensive set that was reduced by backwards elimination to establish potential confounding variables for subsequent specific analyses of height.

Representative and inner-city samples 1987–1988

The main analysis of variables associated with children's height was carried out separately for the representative English and Scottish samples, and the inner-city samples, using the 1987 and 1988 data. The analyses confirmed our previous reports that the variables most strongly related to a child's height were parents' heights, the child's birthweight, and family size (Table 6.1). A difference of 10 cm in maternal or paternal height was associated with a difference in height between 0.3 and

Table 6.2 Height by family size and ethnic background

	Mean height (standard error) (SDS)				
Family size	Representative samples		Inner-city sample		
	England	Scotland	White	Afro-Caribbean	Indian subcontinent
1	0.260 (0.051)	0.117 (0.061)	0.180 (0.091)	0.526 (0.138)	−0.123 (0.213)
2	0.067 (0.020)	0.051 (0.025)	−0.121 (0.048)	0.619 (0.114)	−0.036 (0.078)
3	−0.014 (0.028)	−0.087 (0.033)	−0.311 (0.057)	0.468 (0.119)	−0.309 (0.063)
4	−0.082 (0.046)	−0.244 (0.055)	−0.316 (0.074)	0.511 (0.139)	−0.231 (0.074)
⩾ 5	−0.007 (0.061)	−0.171 (0.086)	−0.522 (0.096)	0.438 (0.154)	−0.374 (0.058)

Taken from Gulliford *et al.*, *Archives of Disease in Childhood*, 1991, **66**, 234–40; with permission from the *BMJ* Publishing Group.

0.5 SDS, equivalent to 2–3 cm in 8-year-old children. Differences in birthweight and length of pregnancy also had a large impact on the height of children. The negative effects in Table 6.1 for length of pregnancy indicate that birthweight overpredicts child's height for full-term pregnancies. The analysis also confirmed that the father's social class was not associated with their child's height after adjustment for the more important factors. Family size was highly associated with children's height in the representative samples, but in the inner-city sample there was an interaction between ethnic group and family size on children's height. The negative association between the number of children in the family and a child's height was shown in white groups in all three samples. However, this association was not demonstrated in the Afro-Caribbeans or children originating from the Indian subcontinent (Table 6.2). In the inner-city sample, children entitled to free school meals were approximately 0.13 SDS shorter than children whose parents paid for school meals. There was little difference between employed mothers and housewives, but unemployed mothers had shorter children in the representative sample (Table 6.1). In 1987–88 English children were still significantly taller than Scottish children, but the difference was equivalent to just 0.3 cm, while in 1972 the difference was 2.0 cm.

Inner-city sample 1983

In the first analysis of data from the inner-city sample (Rona and Chinn 1986) father's unemployment ($p < 0.01$) and mother working outside the home ($p < 0.05$) were associated with a child's height. On average, a child whose father was unemployed was shorter and those with a mother working outside the home taller than other children. A father's social class was not associated with their child's height. In a separate analysis, not including the father's social class or employment status, overall the mother's education was not associated with her child's height, although it was within some of the ethnic groups ($p < 0.05$).

Representative samples 1972

In the first analysis, a father's social class (only in England) and his employment status (only in Scotland) were also associated with height ($p < 0.05$ and $p < 0.01$) in a multiple regression analysis adjusting for parental heights, birthweight, and mother's age (Rona *et al.* 1978). In the analysis based on the 1987 and 1988 data, a father's social class was not associated with his child's height before or after adjustment for parental height, child's birthweight, family size, birth order, and country of residence. A significant interaction between family size and social class on height was found in 1972. In the English sample the height of children in manual classes decreased with an increasing number of children in the family, but this was only seen in the largest families in children in non-manual classes. This interaction was not found in subsequent analyses.

Height and social class

We have been surprised by the weak association between a father's social class and his child's height over the period of the study. Even in 1972, after adjustment for other significant variables in the model, a father's social class only explained 0.1% of the variation in height while the total model explained between 25% and 30% of the variation of height between children. Critical comments have been made about the suitability of adjusting for parental height, on the basis that a father's height is dependent on genes and his own social environment. The majority of studies in developed countries have demonstrated a very high association between parental and child's height (Rona 1981), and most assessing the contribution of genes on children's height (for example twin studies) have shown this to be a substantial factor (Wilson 1979). It is possible that the association between parental and child's height may be inflated by a shared environment of generations. However, a small contribution of father's social class to height was reported by Goldstein (1971) in the 1958 birth cohort study, but the association has decreased over time in the NSHG. This is in contrast to the marked association between the heights of parents and offspring, and indicates that the impact of father's social class on height was already small in 1972 and may have decreased further over time. Even in adults, the 1991 Health Survey for England showed a difference of only 1.6 cm between non-manual and manual social classes (White et al. 1993). As participants in that study were between 16 and 65 years, the result represents the impact of the social environment between 10 and 55 years ago, but this represents the maximum contribution of social class, without adjustment for their birthweight or parental heights.

Other social factors

In the NSHG a large number of sociodemographic factors have been investigated. With the exception of the mother's age at delivery and the number of children in the family the remaining factors have not been associated with height, or inconsistently. In the case of a mother's age at her child's delivery we were inclined to interpret the association with child's height as being unrelated to social factors, since the relationship was not restricted to mothers younger than 20 years of age. In relation to the association between the number of children in the family and height we first thought that the association reflected an effect of social environment, especially in the analysis based on 1972 data, because the association was more noticeable in children whose parents had a manual occupation (Rona et al. 1978). However, it is curious that in subsequent analyses the association has been consistently observed only in white children and not in ethnic minorities. This suggests that cultural characteristics influencing the number of children in the family vary according to ethnicity. In the non-white groups the number of children may be related to social prestige rather than poverty, while in whites it may be more associated with poverty.

Social factors are still associated with a child's height in modern Britain. Entitlement to free school meals, father's unemployment, maternal employment, and the number of children in the family have all been found to be associated in some of our analyses. However, the level to which they are associated with height is small in comparison to factors related to genes or uterine environment—represented in our study by parental heights, ethnic group, birthweight, and length of pregnancy.

Analysis of specific social factors and child's height

In two papers we reported specific analyses on the relation between parents' unemployment status and their child's height (Rona and Chinn 1984a; Rona and Chinn 1991). At the time of the analyses there was public concern over the possible health effects of unemployment, especially in relation to nutritional status. In the 1991 paper we demonstrated that a child whose father was unemployed was shorter, especially if he was unemployed for more than 12 months. The difference, after adjustment for the main factors associated with height, was approximately 1.2 cm. We also looked at height gain over a 2-year period, but we could not show a difference between children according to employment status using change in height SDS between the two occasions. We concluded that the most likely explanation for our findings was that a child was most vulnerable at preschool age to an effect of unemployment on height. Over the period of the study we included the father's employment status in most analyses of height, but the levels of association were inconsistent.

The increasing rates of illegitimacy and divorce over the study period has resulted in a substantial increase in one-parent families, mostly mother-headed families. For this reason we assessed the possible effect of this variable on child's height (Garman et al. 1982), using 1977 data. Although children from one-parent families were slightly shorter than other children, after adjustment for other social factors the mean difference in height between one- and two-parent families was not statistically significant. Our interpretation of the finding was that the growth of children brought up in one-parent families is not jeopardized. In analyses of data from other years one-parent family status was seldom significantly associated with a child's height after adjustment for other social factors.

We also explored the association between vegetarianism and child's height (Rona et al. 1987), and between population density and child's height (Foster et al. 1983). The main group of vegetarians in Britain are of Indian subcontinent origin. Children who were vegetarians in these groups were shorter than children in the same ethnic group who were non-vegetarians. However, the differences were small and not significant ($p > 0.05$) after adjustment, with the exception of that for Urdu girls. Children living in more densely populated parts of Britain were slightly shorter after adjustment for other factors. The difference in height was small and disappeared after adjustment for latitude, which indicates that the finding was related to conditions of living associated with geographical location.

Childhood illness, parents' health-related behaviours, and height

Using data from two surveys, 1973 and 1984, we analysed the association between respiratory illness and height (Rona and Florey 1980; Somerville and Rona 1993). In the second analysis the only variable associated with a child's height, after full adjustment, was wheeze. Children with persistent wheeze were approximately 0.2 SDS shorter than other children. The analyses showed that the difference increased when children who had suffered asthma attacks in the last 12 months were excluded. In 1984, the number of asthma attacks was not associated with a child's height, but it had been in 1973. This could indicate that parents reported milder asthma attacks in their child in the more recent survey, or that children with asthma attacks in 1984 were managed appropriately in contrast to asthmatic children in 1973. In support of the second explanation is the finding in another analysis that approximately 80% of children with asthma attacks were receiving suitable treatment, while only 20% of children with wheeze most days were receiving appropriate treatment (Duran-Tauleria et al. 1996). Frequent cough was significantly related to a child's height in both analyses. However, the difference disappeared after adjustment had been made for other variables. This indicates that children who cough are more likely to belong to groups in society who are shorter, but which factor affects height is difficult to disentangle in this type of analysis.

Height gain and social factors

In an early paper we analysed the association between social factors and height gain from 1972 to 1973 (Smith *et al.* 1980). The analysis involved three types of assessment: final height adjusted for initial height in centimetres; height gain in centimetres; and relative changes in position in terms of the difference between height SDS between the two years. The social variables analysed were family size, father's social class, and whether the father was employed or unemployed. There were very few consistent significant differences in height gain. Change in SDS increased with an increasing number of children in the family. This trend was greater in children in the age range 8 to 10 years than in those aged 5 to 7 years. The results indicated that observed height differences between 5- and 10-year-old children living under different social conditions are largely established before the age of five and do not alter appreciably during primary school years, with some narrowing of the relative family size differences.

Conclusions

Parental heights, child's birthweight, ethnic background, and maternal age at the child's delivery are the variables most consistently related to the height of 5–11-year-old children. Parental height alone explains approximately 15% of the variation in child's height and all the contributing variables in our analyses, including parents' heights, explained between 25% and 30% of the total variation in height. Family size is highly associated with height, but only in white children. Social class as assessed by the father's occupation does not make an independent contribution to the variation in height. Several other social variables, such as father's employment status and maternal employment, are inconsistently related to a child's height. The associations were found in some of the analyses or in some of the samples. Children with a persistent wheeze were shorter. Rates of growth over a 1- or 2-year period were rarely associated with any social variable in the study. This shows that height differences related to social factors were established before the child entered primary school. In Britain today, genes and the maternal environment are the factors most strongly related to a child's height, while social factors are only marginally related to a child's height with the exception of family size in white children.

7 Factors related to obesity

Background

Overweight and obesity in primary school children were considered only ancillary information by the Sub-committee on Nutritional Surveillance in its first report (Department of Health and Social Security 1973). The Sub-committee endorsed the measurement of weight and, without much enthusiasm, the measurement of skinfold thickness. The marked increase in obesity in the last 20 years in several European countries (Colhoun and Prescott-Clarke 1996; Hughes *et al*. 1997; Kuskowska-Wolk and Bergstrom 1993; Sorensen and Price 1990), and in the US (Gortmaker *et al*. 1987; Troiano *et al*. 1995), has focused attention on four areas: the possible causes of obesity in childhood; the possible effects of obesity in childhood and on adult morbidity; the risk of obese children becoming obese adults; and the search for the effective prevention and treatment of obesity. The concern that once a child is obese it is at increased risk of becoming an obese adult has added interest to the study of child obesity, although the association between child and adult obesity has been shown to be only moderate (Lake *et al*. 1997; Serdula *et al*. 1993). The evidence that obese adults have increased mortality—and also that adult obesity is associated with non-insulin-dependent diabetes, osteoarthritis, high blood pressure, and hyperlipidaemia as well as ovarian, endometrial, and breast cancer—places the study of childhood obesity in a priority area for research (Scottish Intercollegiate Guidelines Network 1996). The relative scarcity of effective and affordable interventions into obesity in children gives further stimulus to efforts aimed at understanding the social and behavioural mechanisms involved in the aetiology of obesity.

The NSHG has contributed to the identification of factors associated with overweight and obesity. It has also contributed to the assessment of the possible effects of obesity on other CHD (Coronary heart disease) risk factors and respiratory illness in children. These two aspects will be reviewed below. It is important to understand the relationship between the two proxy measures of obesity used in our study, weight-for-height and triceps skinfold, before considering our findings. We also comment on the merits of using BIA (bioelectrical impedance analysis) in epidemiological studies in children.

Weight-for-height, skinfold thickness, and BIA

Triceps skinfold thickness was measured in all surveys of the study. In the last 6 years of the study we also measured subscapular skinfold. Suprailiac and biceps skinfold thicknesses were measured, only in 9-year-old children, in the last 3 years of the study. The suitability of indices of weight-for-height to assess adiposity in childhood has been discussed frequently. Morris and Chinn (1981) assessed the relation of weight-to-height and triceps skinfold thickness. They demonstrated that height and triceps skinfold explained approximately 75% of the variation in weight, but over the 5- to 11-year age range the partial regression coefficient on height decreased, while that on triceps skinfold almost doubled in both sexes. This finding may be related to the increase of fat near to puberty and it serves as a cautionary note over the interpretation of weight-for-height in childhood at different ages. Morris and Chinn (1981) also assessed the correlation between weight-for-height and triceps skinfold. There was an increase of the correlation from around 0.5 at 5 years of age to

0.7 at age 11, again demonstrating that an index of weight-for-height reflects adiposity in the prepubertal period more appropriately than in younger children. The study was helpful for also illustrating the difficulty of defining obesity consistently in this age range. Only half the children with a weight-for-height above the 90th centile had a triceps skinfold above the 90th centile. This suggests that a large number of children may be heavy, but not obese. It also may explain why some factors described below are associated with one of the proxy measurements of adiposity, but not with the other. Of more relevance for monitoring obesity is that the two measurements provide different information, as shown in the USA where, using the same data set, one group assessing skinfold thickness (Gortmaker et al. 1987) reported an increase in obesity and another assessing weight-for-height (Harlan et al. 1988) reported no increase.

There has been interest in the use of BIA in epidemiological studies for its simplicity and low cost. In theory body impedance is negatively related to body volume, and using this relation it is possible to estimate TBW (total body water). TBW can be used to derive FFM (fat free mass) and hence body fat from the FFM and weight. We piloted the use of BIA in the NSHG as an alternative measure of obesity to that of skinfold thickness in 77 children (Hammond et al. 1994b). We assessed the repeatability of the sum of skinfolds at four sites and BIA, and their agreement in estimating body fat. Both measurements were highly repeatable. However, the level of agreement between body fat estimates from prediction equations based on skinfolds thickness or impedance measurements was poor. Measurements of body fat derived from BIA were moderately correlated with the weight-for-height index, but less than that of any of the skinfold measurements. Our conclusion was that until BIA measurements are shown to be related to cardiovascular disease, or studies in children show that a good measure of fat can be derived from BIA (regardless of gender, age, and ethnicity), it is unwise to replace skinfold measurements by BIA in community studies.

Factors related to obesity

We have published three papers assessing the main factors associated with weight-for-height and triceps skinfold (Duran-Tauleria et al. 1995; Rona and Chinn 1982a, 1987a). In the paper by Duran-Tauleria and colleagues (1995) subscapular skinfold was also assessed. In the two first analyses weight-for-height was calculated as weight SDS adjusted for height SDS, and in the third analysis as $\log_{10}[(\text{weight} - 9)/\text{height}^{3.7}]$, an index independent of age and sex (Chinn et al. 1992). The analysis published in 1982 was based on the English and Scottish representative samples, the paper published in 1987 reported the findings in the inner-city sample, and in 1995 we reported findings in the three samples using data collected in 1990 and 1991. We will describe the findings in the last analysis and report details from previous analyses. In all the analyses, unless otherwise stated, the associations described are those that were associated with the dependent variable, at least at the conventional statistical significance level of 5%.

Table 7.1 shows the main factors associated with weight-for-height in the 1990/91 analysis. Parental BMI (body mass index) assessed from reported height and weight was highly associated with the child's weight-for-height ($p < 0.001$). A significant interaction of ethnic origin and family size on weight-for-height was found. There was no indication that maternal BMI was more strongly related to the child's weight-for-height than paternal BMI. Children in one-parent families were more likely to be overweight, especially in the rare case of the father being the single parent ($p = 0.002$). Mothers working more than 25 hours per week outside the home had heavier children ($p = 0.02$). Birthweight was positively associated with child's weight-for-height, but a significant interaction indicated that the slope of the association was less steep in older than younger children in the analysis ($p = 0.004$). The variables significantly associated with children's weight-for-height explained 13% of the variation.

Table 7.1 Variables associated with weight-for-height index

Variable	Coefficient (SE)	p Value
Mother's BMI (kg/m^2)	0.049 (0.002)	< 0.001
Father's BMI (kg/m^2)	0.068 (0.003)	< 0.001
Birthweight and age interaction		0.004
Birthweight (kg) (<7 years)	0.309 (0.048)	
Difference in slope from<7 years group		
7–8 years	0.004 (0.061)	
8–10 years	−0.135 (0.060)	
>10 years	−0.153 (0.063)	
Parenting		0.002
Both parents at home	0	
Only mother at home	0.102 (0.033)	
Only father at home	0.337 (0.137)	
Neither at home	0.057 (0.100)	
Mother's hours of work		0.02
>25 hours per week	0	
15–25 hours per week	−0.050 (0.034)	
<15 hours per week	−0.085 (0.038)	
No work outside home	−0.104 (0.031)	
Unknown	−0.052 (0.094)	

Ethnic group and family size interaction $p = 0.019$.
Taken from Duran-Tauleria *et al.*, *Journal of Epidemiology and Community Health*, 1995, **49**, 466–73, with permission from the *BMJ* Publishing Group.

Analyses, including the same independent variables, were carried out in relation to children's triceps and subscapular skinfold thickness, separately and in summation. The results were similar, so that only the associations with the sum of skinfolds are given (Table 7.2). Parental BMI, the child's birthweight, and the mother's age at her child's delivery were associated with the outcome variable ($p < 0.001$). Only 8% of the variation in skinfold thickness was explained by the variables in the model.

Logistic regression analysis was used to assess the factors associated with obesity, as defined by the upper quartile of the distribution of weight-for-height. Children were divided into two groups: those in the upper quartile of the distribution and the rest. Most of the factors related to the outcome measure in the multiple linear regression of weight-for-height were also statistically significant in the logistic regression analysis, but the father's social class was also associated with the outcome variable, although weakly. A child was 3.5 times more likely to be in the upper quartile of weight-for-height if both parents were in the upper quartile of BMI and twice as likely if one parent was in the upper quartile of the distribution (Fig. 7.1). An only child tended to be heavier than children with siblings, and was between 1.66 and three times more likely to be in the upper quartile of the distribution than those in families with four or more sibs (Fig. 7.2). Likewise a child in a one-parent family had a higher risk of being heavier, especially if the parent was a father (Fig. 7.3).

In a similar analysis in relation to skinfold thickness, the logistic regression showed that a child whose parent's BMIs were in the upper quartile, whose birthweight was in the upper quartile, who

Table 7.2 Variables associated with $\log_{10}$(sum of subscapular and triceps skinfold thickness)

Variable	Coefficient (SE)	p Value
Mother's BMI (kg/m^2)	0.078 (0.005)	< 0.001
Father's BMI (kg/m^2)	0.087 (0.006)	< 0.001
Birthweight (kg)	0.256 (0.036)	< 0.001
Mother's age at child's birth	0.013 (0.002)	< 0.001
Drinks milk at school		0.01
Yes	0	
No	0.055 (0.023)	
Unknown	0.140 (0.056)	

Ethnic group and family size interaction $p = 0.005$.
Taken from Duran-Tauleria *et al.*, *Journal of Epidemiology and Community Health*, 1995, **49**, 466–73, with permission from the *BMJ* Publishing Group.

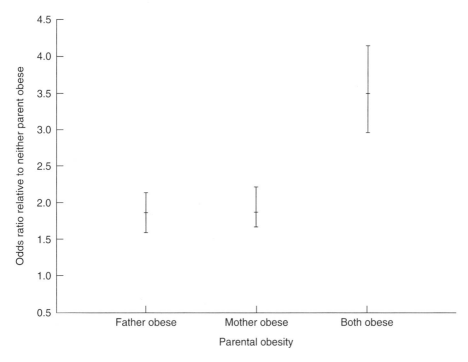

Fig. 7.1 Odds ratio and 95% confidence interval of a child being in the upper quartile of weight-for-height by number of parents in the upper quartile of body mass index (BMI), relative to no parent in the upper quartile. Results taken from Duran-Tauleria *et al.*, *Journal of Epidemiology and Community Health*, 1995, **49**, 466–73; with permission from the *BMJ* Publishing Group.

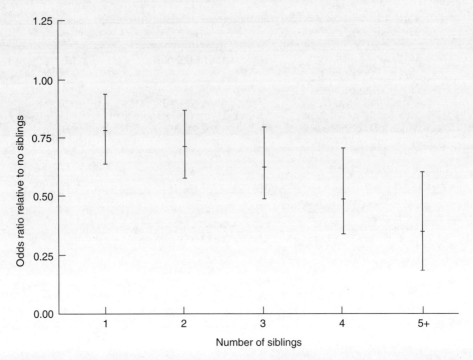

Fig. 7.2   Odds ratio and 95% confidence interval of a child being in the upper quartile of weight-for-height by number of siblings, relative to no sibling. Results taken from Duran-Tauleria *et al.*, *Journal of Epidemiology and Community Health*, 1995, **49**, 466–73; with permission from the *BMJ* Publishing Group.

had an older mother at child's birth, was the only child in the family, or whose mother worked outside the home was more likely to be in the upper quartile of the skinfold distribution. Scottish, Urdu, and Punjabi children were also more likely to have higher levels of adiposity.

   In the analysis carried out for each ethnic group it was found that the level of association between parents' height and weight with child's weight-for-height and triceps skinfold varied according to ethnic group (Rona and Chinn 1987a). As parents' weights and heights were recorded, and not measured, the variation may be due to a genuine difference between groups, but it may also be due to bias in the level of the accuracy of the information between ethnic groups. In a small validation study of information on height we found that for Asian mothers, but not fathers, the differences between reported and measured heights were larger than in any other ethnic group (Rona *et al.* 1989). In white fathers we also detected a large difference between recorded and measured height, although it did not reach statistical significance level in a very small sample. Rona and Chinn (1987a) also found that there were large differences in triceps skinfold thickness between ethnic groups. Afro-Caribbean children, although of similar weight-for-height to white children, had a substantially lower median triceps skinfold. Chinn and colleagues (1992) also assessed the differences between ethnic groups of BMI, weight-for-height index, and the sum of triceps and subscapular skinfolds, using data from the 1989 and 1990 surveys. The mean weight-for-height index showed that all groups originating from the Indian subcontinent were lighter than children from other ethnic groups (Table 7.3). Afro-Caribbean children were markedly thinner than white children, as measured by total skinfold thickness, despite being slightly heavier than white children

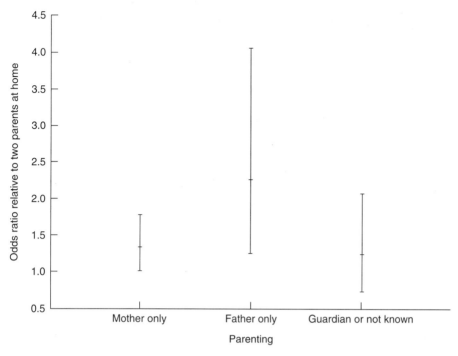

Fig. 7.3 Odds ratio and 95% confidence interval of a child being in the upper quartile of weight-for-height by number of parents at home, relative to two parents at home. Results taken from Duran-Tauleria *et al.*, *Journal of Epidemiology and Community Health*, 1995, **49**, 466–73; with permission from the *BMJ* Publishing Group.

Table 7.3 Mean and standard deviation (SD) of weight-for-height and total skinfold (triceps plus subscapular skinfolds) by ethnic group in units of standard deviation score (SDS)

	Boys		Girls	
	Weight-for-height (SDS) Mean (SD)	Total skinfold (SDS) Mean (SD)	Weight-for-height (SDS) Mean (SD)	Total skinfold (SDS) Mean (SD)
White (England representative)	0.00 (1.00)	0.00 (0.97)	0.01 (1.00)	0.00 (098)
White (Scotland representative)	0.04 (1.03)	0.10 (0.98)***	−0.01 (0.24)	−0.05 (0.98)
White (England inner city)	0.02 (1.00)	0.10 (0.89)***	−0.04 (1.00)	−0.02 (0.97)
Afro-Caribbean	0.04 (1.05)	−0.28 (1.02)***	0.04 (1.10)	−0.30 (1.19)***
Urdu	−0.41 (1.28)***	0.22 (1.11)***	−0.45 (1.17)***	0.11 (1.02)
Gujarati	−0.88 (1.23)***	−0.23 (1.15)***	−0.87 (1.12)***	−0.35 (1.10)***
Punjabi	−0.42 (1.32)***	0.12 (1.10)**	−0.56 (1.10)***	−0.12 (1.05)**
Other Indian	−0.33 (1.37)***	−0.04 (1.22)	−0.60 (1.13)***	−0.23 (1.09)*

Significance of difference of mean from that of English representative sample. $^*p < 0.05$; $^{**}p < 0.01$; $^{***}p < 0.001$.
Taken from Chinn *et al.*1992, with permission.

(Table 7.3). Except for the Urdu-speaking group, girls of Indian subcontinent origin were thinner than white English girls, but Urdu- and Punjabi-speaking boys were significantly fatter than white boys.

The results described above demonstrated that, after ethnicity, parental BMI is the most important factor associated with a child's adiposity. This association could be explained as an inherited susceptibility in children, as suggested by twin studies (Bodhurta *et al.* 1990). As families share an environment it is also possible that part of the association between parents and children may be related to physical activity and diet within families. However, the lack of difference in the correlation of BMI between twins reared apart and those reared together provides strong evidence that the within-family association of obesity is mediated through a genetic mechanism rather than an environmental mechanism (Stunkard *et al.* 1990).

The health implications of the association between birthweight and child obesity is not straightforward. Barker *et al.* (1992*a*) have reported that low birthweight is associated with coronary heart disease mortality. However, an overweight child is more likely to become an overweight adult and have a higher risk of hypertension, high cholesterol levels, and low physical fitness. The issue is further complicated by the finding in the Dutch famine study that those individuals whose mother starved in the first half of their gestation during the Second World War were more likely to become obese in adult life (Ravelli *et al.* 1976).

Although sociodemographic factors were not major factors in explaining the variability of weight-for-height, our analyses indicate that several factors within families may increase the risk of a child's obesity. The fact that children in a one-parent family, those whose mother worked outside the home for more than 25 hours per week, and those who were an only child were more likely to be obese, may indicate that children who spend long periods of time on their own may be more at risk. Possible explanations for these findings are overprotection of children under these circumstances, lack of supervision, or lack of stimulation. Our findings are consistent with the reported association between time spent watching television and the level of fatness (Andersen *et al.* 1998). Social factors, which are intended to measure social disadvantage such as father's occupation or employment status, were not associated with weight-for-height in most analyses. This is in contrast with our finding in an analysis of data for parents of children in our study, in which there was an association between father's social class and parental weight for height, especially in mothers (Rona and Morris 1982). In the 1995 Health Survey for England it was also reported that social class is more highly associated with obesity in women than in men (White *et al.* 1993).

Weight-for-height and skinfold thickness as independent factors

We investigated the association of weight-for-height and skinfold thickness with CHD risk factors (Bettiol *et al.* 1999; Kikuchi *et al.* 1995; Rona *et al.* 1996) in 9-year-old children, and also in relation to respiratory symptoms in the total sample (Somerville *et al.* 1984). These aspects are covered more extensively in Chapter 8 for CHD and in Chapter 9 for respiratory illness. In summary, adiposity, as measured by weight-for-height or the sum of skinfold thickness measured at four sites (suprailiac, triceps, biceps, and subscapular), was consistently and highly associated with systolic and diastolic blood pressure, total serum cholesterol, and cardiorespiratory fitness ($p < 0.001$). Children who were fatter were more likely to have high total cholesterol, high systolic and diastolic blood pressure (Rona *et al.* 1996), and poor physical fitness (Bettiol *et al.* 1999; Kikuchi *et al.* 1995). Similar findings have been also reported by others (Armstrong *et al.* 1990; Burns *et al.* 1989; Freedman *et al.* 1987; Lauer *et al.* 1991; Szklo 1979; Webber *et al.* 1991). In relation to physical fitness the worrying aspect of the association is that obesity and low physical activity enhance each other. Obese children are less likely to embark on strenuous physical activity and children who do not exercise are more likely to become obese.

Children with wheeze, bronchitis attacks or asthma attacks, and colds going to the chest had a greater weight-for-height and triceps skinfold. Cross-sectional analyses do not determine the direction of the relation. Children with respiratory illness may be less willing to exercise, but it is also possible that obese children have an increasing susceptibility to respiratory illness. In adults, there are reports of an association between obesity and respiratory illness (Negri *et al.* 1988; Seidell *et al.* 1986; Shaheen *et al.* 1999).

Conclusions

Childhood obesity has become an area of concern because of the increase in adiposity shown in adults and children in the Western world. Parental BMI is the variable most strongly positively associated with a child's weight-for-height and skinfold thickness in the NSHG. A child's birthweight is also highly associated with proxy measures of obesity, but the level of association declines with the age of the child. There are large differences in triceps skinfold thickness between ethnic groups, with the Afro-Caribbean group being leanest despite having similar weight-for-height to that of the white children. Children in one-parent families, those who are the only child in the family, and those whose mother work outside the home for more than 25 hours a week have higher adiposity than other children. Our findings indicate that genetic endowment, some aspect of shared family environment, and social factors related to children spending long hours without company are risk factors for obesity in childhood. Although overt pathology related to obesity is rare in childhood, children with higher weight-for-height or skinfold thickness are less physically fit, have higher total cholesterol and blood pressure level, and have a higher prevalence of asthma symptoms than other children.

8 Coronary heart disease risk factors in children

Background

By 1990 there was growing interest in the study of coronary heart disease (CHD) risk factors in British children. Britain is one of the countries with the highest CHD mortality in the world (Kesteloot and Joossens 1992). Information on CHD risk factors in children was limited, so a study of these was essential given the worrying increase in obesity in children (Chinn and Rona 1987a, 1994; Chinn et al. 1998a; Hughes et al. 1997). Although blood pressure in children had been studied in large community samples in Britain (De Swiet et al. 1992; Holland and Beresford 1974; Law et al. 1993; Whincup et al. 1992), this was not the case for serum cholesterol levels in the community, for which few data were available (Boreham et al. 1993; Sporik et al. 1991). This was in contrast to the USA and many other countries (Cresanta et al. 1982; Knuiman et al. 1980; Resnicow et al. 1989). Knuiman and colleagues (1980) demonstrated a large variation in total cholesterol levels in 7- to 9-year-olds between countries, and these differences broadly corresponded to variations in CHD mortality rates. Information on physical fitness in prepubertal children was also scarce in Britain. Blood pressure and cholesterol level were included in the NSHG in 1992 after piloting these procedures in several schools in Bath, and also that for cholesterol in adults of the Department of Public Health Medicine at St Thomas'. Physical fitness tests were also piloted in schools in Bath and Birmingham. We would have liked to assess physical activity as well as physical fitness, but at the time of the study we were unconvinced that questions on physical activity in children were sufficiently valid, and other types of measurement within the NSHG framework were considered unfeasible. The assessment of physical fitness is particularly important because it has been reported that levels of physical activity in British children are poor (Armstrong et al. 1990). The cycle-ergometer test was included in the study in 1992. The NSHG is the only study that can provide information on CHD risk factors in the main ethnic groups in Britain.

Measurements

Blood pressure, cholesterol level, and physical fitness were assessed in children in classes in which the majority would be 9 years of age by the end of the school year. Blood pressure was measured using the Dinamap 1846 automated sphygmomanometer on the right arm. A small adult-size cuff was used to take three blood pressure measurements at 1-minute intervals and the mean of the three measurements used for analysis.

The cholesterol concentration in capillary blood was measured in 1992 and 1993 using the Lipotrend C, a portable reflectance photometer. The fieldworker gently squeezed the child's finger filling a capillary tube as recommended. In 1994, after an extensive pilot study in several schools in Canterbury (Hammond et al. 1994a, 1994c), venepuncture sessions were introduced in the English representative sample and in one-third of the Scottish representative areas. Tubes of blood were sent by first-class post to the Chemical Pathology Laboratory at Guy's Hospital, London. Serum cholesterol was measured using a Kodak Ektachem Chemistry Slide (CHOL) and high-density lipoproteins (HDL)-cholesterol using the Kodak Ektachem HDL-cholesterol kit.

Physical fitness was measured using the cycle-ergometer test in 1992 and 1993. PWC85%, power output against load at 85% of the maximum heart rate, was measured to assess physical fitness. The cycle-ergometer was standardized for adolescents by Eurofit (Committee for the Development of Sport 1988). Based on several pilot studies the test was modified to suit 9-year-olds. PWC85% in adolescents corresponds to a pulse rate of 170/min, while in 9-year-olds it corresponds to approximately 185/min. In the first pilot study we followed the Eurofit protocol in every detail, but we needed to stop the test because most 9-year-olds reached a pulse rate above 170/min at an early stage of the assessment. In the test the child was asked to ride the cycle for 6 minutes and the load was increased every 2 minutes according to the child's pulse rate in the last 10 seconds of each 2-minute period. Children were stopped if their pulse rate reached 196/min or if they became too exhausted. If the pre-established heart rate was not reached at the end of the 6 minutes the test was continued for another 2 minutes with an increased fourth load. PWC85% was calculated using the data at the last two loads by linear interpolation (Kikuchi et al. 1995).

The three measurements required positive parental consent and the willingness of the child to participate—Chapter 3 gives details. The children were keen to participate in the cycle-ergometer test, but less so to provide a blood sample.

Cholesterol level

The data on total cholesterol, HDL-cholesterol, and other constituents, measured in 1994 have provided an estimation of 95% reference ranges for blood constituents (Chinn et al. 1998b). Analyses of the factors associated with raised cholesterol levels used the measurements from the Lipotrend C in the 1992 and 1993 surveys (Rona et al. 1996). Table 8.1 shows the variables found to be significantly associated, at least at the 5% level. The sum of skinfold thickness, measured at four sites (triceps, biceps, suprailiac, and subscapular), was highly and positively associated with total cholesterol ($p < 0.001$). Height was highly and negatively associated with total cholesterol ($p < 0.001$). Ethnic background was strongly related to total cholesterol ($p < 0.001$); some of the groups originating from the Indian subcontinent had high cholesterol levels (Punjabi and the heterogeneous group of Others from the Indian subcontinent), but Urdu and Gujarati children had low cholesterol levels. White children in inner-city areas had higher cholesterol levels than other white children. Only children had higher cholesterol levels than children with siblings ($p = 0.03$) and girls had higher cholesterol levels than boys ($p = 0.03$).

Measurements based on the Lipotrend C were consistent and repeatable, but they underestimated total cholesterol values in comparison to determinations made by the Chemical Pathology Laboratory at Guy's Hospital. Table 8.2 gives the mean and 95% range of total and HDL cholesterol for 9-year-old children based on the laboratory determinations. Total cholesterol was significantly higher in girls than in boys by 3.3% ($p = 0.003$). The 95% range included values above 5.2 mmol/l which are above the recommended level in adults (Shepherd et al. 1987). In the main survey 8.7% of the children had a cholesterol above 5.2 mmol/l, and in our pilot study in Canterbury 23% of the children were above this value. The implications of these findings need discussion because to include values between 5.2 and 5.79 mmol/l as reference values is inconsistent with prevailing recommendations in adults. However, it is unclear whether management of children with a cholesterol level below 5.8 mmol/l is efficacious and there is uncertainty about the possible damage to the child and family that this action would cause. Knuiman and colleagues (1980) assessed total cholesterol and HDL cholesterol in children of 7 and 8 years, slightly younger than the NSHG children; the means of several European samples were similar to the geometric means in the NSHG. The mean total cholesterol in the Bogalusa Heart Study of 10-year-old children was

Table 8.1   Variables associated with total serum cholesterol (log mmol) as determined by the Lipotrend C

Variable	Coefficient	p Value
Log_{10}(sum of skinfolds)	0.0603	< 0.001
Height (cm)	−0.0013	< 0.001
Gender		0.03
Girls	0	
Boys	−0.0160	
Ethnic origin		< 0.001
White (English representative)	0	
White (Scottish representative)	0.0096	
White (English inner-city)	0.0200	
Afro-Caribbean	0.0231	
Urdu	−0.0032	
Gujarati	−0.0309	
Punjabi	0.0301	
Others (Indian subcontinent)	0.0398	
Others	0.0076	
No. of children in family		0.03
Not known	0	
1	0.0082	
2	−0.0099	
3 or 4	−0.0017	
5 or more	−0.0141	

Taken from Rona *et al.*, *Journal of Epidemiology and Community Health*, 1996, **50**, 512–18; with permission from the *BMJ* Publishing Group.

slightly lower than the geometric mean in the NSHG (Cresanta *et al.* 1982; Gidding *et al.* 1995). These comparisons need to be interpreted with caution as the methods used to assess lipoprotein levels and the summary statistics were different.

Blood pressure

The geometric means and 95% range for systolic and diastolic blood pressure in boys and girls were 109.4 (95% range, 94.2 to 127.3), 57.4 (95% range, 44.3 to 74.4), 110.3 (95% range, 93.5 to 131.3), and 58.0 (95% range, 44.8 to 75.2), respectively. The medians of diastolic and systolic blood pressure levels recently reported for 7–9-year-olds in the 1996 Health Survey for England were similar in both sexes (Dong *et al.* 1998). Height and weight-for-height were highly associated with systolic blood pressure ($p < 0.001$) (Table 8.3). Heavier and taller children had higher blood pressure. Birthweight was weakly associated with systolic blood pressure ($p = 0.03$), but allowing for the birthweight relationship children with a shorter gestation (less than 37 weeks) had higher blood pressure ($p = 0.002$). Although ethnic origin was related to systolic blood pressure ($p = 0.04$) the heterogeneity between groups was small. The significant variables explained 17% of the variation in systolic blood pressure.

Height was also associated with diastolic blood pressure ($p < 0.001$), and with log (sum of skinfolds) rather than with weight-for-height ($p < 0.001$). There were significant associations with diastolic blood pressure of regional health authority ($p = 0.001$), number of children in the family

Table 8.2 Mean and 95% range of total and HDL cholesterol in children between 8 and 10 years (as measured in the Chemical Pathology Laboratory at Guy's Hospital)

Variable	Geometric mean (mmol/l)	95% range (mmol/l)
Total cholesterol	4.32	3.22 to 5.79
Cholesterol (HDL)	1.41	0.90 to 2.10

Taken from Chinn et al. 1998b; with permission.
To convert cholesterol in mmol/l to mg/dl multiply by 38.5.

Table 8.3 Variables associated with systolic blood pressure in 8–10-year-old children

Variable		
Coefficient	p Value	
Height (cm)	0.0014	< 0.001
Weight-for-height index	0.1262	< 0.001
Birthweight (kg)	−0.0041	0.03
Length of gestation		0.002
⩽ 37 weeks	0.0083	
⩾ 38 weeks	0.0001	
Not known	0	
Ethnic origin		0.04
White (English representative)		
White (Scottish representative)	0.0026	
White (English inner-city)	−0.0087	
Afro-Caribbean	0.0030	
Urdu	0.0081	
Gujarati	−0.0091	
Punjabi	0.0043	
Other (Indian subcontinent)	0.0073	
Others	0.0004	

Taken from Rona et al., *Journal of Epidemiology and Community Health*, 1996, **50**, 512–18; with permission from the *BMJ* Publishing Group.

($p = 0.009$), and father's social class ($p = 0.003$). Most of these associations seemed chance findings; for social class the group with no information had the highest diastolic blood pressure, the variation between regional health authorities did not show concordance with mortality for coronary heart disease in adults, and for the number of children in the family there was no consistent trend.

The factor most strongly associated with the blood pressure level in our analysis was weight-for-height or skinfold thickness. This had been found in several earlier studies (Lauer et al. 1991; Szklo 1979; Webber et al. 1991). Although we confirmed the association between birthweight and systolic blood pressure previously reported (Barker et al. 1989; Law et al. 1993; Whincup et al. 1989), this association was weaker than the association between weight-for-height and systolic blood pressure.

Adiposity was represented in the analyses by two independent variables: weight-for height and log (skinfold thickness at four sites). In the final model only one of the two variables remained statistically significant. The fact that for systolic blood pressure it was skinfold thickness and for diastolic blood pressure it was weight-for-height may be a consequence of the higher association between weight-for-height and triceps skinfold thickness in 9-year-old children than in younger age groups.

Physical fitness

There have been two papers published in relation to physical fitness in 9-year-old children. Kikuchi *et al.* (1995) analysed data based on the English representative sample and Bettiol *et al.* (1999) studied all three samples. The results were analysed in two ways: by logistic regression analysis to assess factors related to the ability to finish at least 4 minutes of the test (this is the minimum for calculating PWC85%); and using multiple linear regression analysis to estimate effects associated with PWC85%. Using the most recent analysis, which included the three samples (Bettiol *et al.* 1999), the most consistent factors associated with physical fitness were the sum of skinfolds, height, and ethnic group. A child with a total skinfold thickness of 50 mm was around 30% less likely to complete 4 minutes of the test than a child with a total skinfold of 25 mm. Of the children who finished the test there was a strong negative association between skinfold thickness and PWC85% in boys and girls. Taller children were more likely to finish the test and, of those who finished the test, to perform better than smaller children. Children belonging to the Indian subcontinent group were less likely to continue the test for at least 4 minutes and the performance of those whose PWC85% could be estimated was worse, especially in girls, than that of children from other ethnic groups. Approximately one-third of the children from the Indian subcontinent group were unable to finish the test compared to between 10% and 18% of children in other ethnic groups. Other variables were inconsistently associated with physical fitness. There was no indication that children with a less advantageous social background had poorer physical fitness than other children.

Interpretation

Obesity is the main factor consistently and highly associated with most other CHD risk factors in childhood. Weight-for-height and skinfold thickness are easy to measure and relatively easy to interpret in children. Physical activity, blood pressure, and cholesterol assessments in children are either difficult to assess, less acceptable in the community as measurements in healthy children, or have low accuracy. In a comparison of risk factors in children who had a parent with CHD with those who did not, skinfold thickness and body mass index were consistently different between the ages of 10 and 25 years (Bao *et al.* 1997). For cholesterol, blood pressure, glucose levels, and endogenous insulin there were no differences between the two groups in children; differences started to appear in young adults for cholesterol, glucose, and insulin levels, but not blood pressure. As in the NSHG, the Muscatine and the Bogalusa studies in the USA have demonstrated that obese children have higher levels of serum cholesterol than other children (Burns *et al.* 1989; Freedman *et al.* 1987) and in the Bogolusa study fatness was associated with most CHD risk factors in children and young adults (Webber *et al.* 1995). Obesity and smoking behaviour are the two most important health indicators that need to be monitored in British children.

Conclusions

Either weight-for-height or skinfold thickness were highly and positively associated with total cholesterol, systolic and diastolic blood pressure, and physical fitness. Height was also highly associated with both variables, but it was positively associated with blood pressure and negatively associated with total cholesterol. Length of gestation was negatively associated with systolic blood pressure. Children originating in the Indian subcontinent were identified as having poor physical fitness in comparison to other ethnic groups. There were other variables associated with the dependent variables, but the associations were borderline significant or there was no trend between the categories and the dependent variables. Approximately 9% of the children had a cholesterol level above 5.2 mmol/l, considered the upper limit of the recommended range in adults. The most important message emerging from our results is that obesity is associated with most other CHD risk factors in children. Monitoring the levels of fatness in childhood may provide a helpful tool for predicting the risk of CHD in adulthood.

9 Studies on respiratory illness and lung function

Background

Respiratory illness is a major contributor to hospital admissions and readmissions in childhood (Anderson 1989a). There is also some evidence that respiratory illness in childhood may contribute to reduced lung function in adulthood (Shaheen *et al*. 1998). The NSHG provided an opportunity for assessing respiratory symptoms in the community. From 1973 questions on respiratory illness were included in the study, which, with small modifications, were kept over the study period (Table 9.1). Outdoor pollution, SO_2, and smoke, was sampled at each school every 24 hours, and data on indoor pollution, based on the type of fuel used for cooking and the number of people in the home in 1977 who smoked cigarettes, a pipe, or cigars, were collected. The studies on outdoor pollution, on a cross-sectional and a longitudinal basis, were carried out between 1973 and 1977, and were partially able to allay worries in relation to the possible effects of outdoor pollution on respiratory illness. Indeed, during the study period smoke and SO_2 markedly decreased. An association between smoke level and respiratory levels was found, but as the levels of smoke in the study areas were lower than those thought necessary for an effect on respiratory illness the authors concluded that this relation was unlikely to be causal (Melia *et al*. 1981a, b). Over the last 20 years the measurement of small smoke particles, less than 10 μm, and other components in outdoor pollution have been considered important in assessing the health hazards of outdoor pollution (Ashmore 1995). Thus the analysis based on NSHG data contributes little to answering current questions on the relation between outdoor pollution and health. This is in contrast to the finding, first reported from the NSHG, of an association between gas cooking and respiratory illness (Melia *et al*. 1977). Since the publication of this report others have found the relation in children, and more recently in adult women (Jarvis *et al*. 1996; Speizer *et al*. 1980; Volkmer *et al*. 1995).

The NSHG has contributed to our knowledge in relation to several other issues of respiratory illness. Over the study period new measurements were included for a short period, such as lung function and exercise-induced bronchial responsiveness (see Chapter 2), and in the questionnaire new items were added such as medication for children with respiratory illness. These additions to the study have allowed us to contribute to a large number of topics in addition to the indoor and outdoor air pollution studies. The effect of parental smoking on lung function and respiratory

Table 9.1   Questions on respiratory symptoms and illness in the NSHG

Has he or she suffered from either of the following illnesses in the last 12 months?
   Asthma. If yes, how many attacks in the last 12 months?
   Bronchitis. If yes, how many attacks in the last 12 months?
Does he or she usually cough first thing in the morning (excluding clearing throat or single cough)?
Does he or she usually cough at any other time (excluding clearing throat or single cough)?
Does his or her chest ever sound wheezy or whistling?
   If yes, does he or she get this on most days or nights?
Do colds go to his or her chest?

Table 9.2   Prevalence of respiratory illness or symptoms by ethnic background and sample

	Representative samples		Inner-city sample		
	England (%)	Scotland (%)	White (%)	Afro-Caribbean (%)	Indian subcontinent (%)
Any respiratory symptom	29.7	27.9	41.9	50.6	29.0
Persistent wheeze with or without asthma attacks	6.8	5.4	9.2	9.1	6.1
Asthma attacks	5.3	4.0	4.6	5.0	3.8
Number of children	5616	3814	1688	678	1985

Duran-Tauleria *et al*. The results were first published in the *BMJ* (Influence of ethnic group on asthma treatment in children in 1990–1; national cross sectional study. *British Medical Journal*, 1996, **313**, 148–52) and are reproduced by permission of the *BMJ*.

illness, the secular trend of asthma in England and Scotland, and the prevalence of food intolerance, including food allergy, are described in other chapters of the book.

In this chapter we describe the differences in respiratory illness and lung function according to ethnicity in Britain, the association between respiratory illness and anthropometric measurements, aetiological factors related to respiratory illness, and social inequalities in relation to the distribution of asthma and its management in the community.

Respiratory illness and lung function according to ethnic group

Of the large community studies in Britain the NSHG is the only one that has included a large sample of children from ethnic minorities. We studied the prevalence of respiratory illness in the main ethnic groups in Britain in two analyses (Duran-Tauleria *et al*. 1996; Melia *et al*. 1988). We also studied the differences in FEV_1 (forced expiratory volume in one second), FVC (forced vital capacity), FEF_{25-75} (forced expiratory flow rate between 25% and 75% of FVC), and FEF_{75-85} (forced expiratory flow rate between 75% and 85% of FVC) in the same ethnic groups (Chinn and Rona 1992). While the results on respiratory symptoms are based on the total sample, lung function results were confined to children between the ages of 7 and 11 years as the proportion of satisfactory measurements decreases sharply below the age of 7.

The two analyses assessing the prevalence of respiratory illness, one based on 1982 and 1983 English data (Melia *et al*. 1988) and the other on 1990 and 1991 data including all three samples (Duran-Tauleria *et al*. 1996), showed similar results. Respiratory illnesses were more frequent in whites and Afro-Caribbean children in inner-city areas, and lowest in whites in the representative samples and in those from the Indian subcontinent (Table 9.2). Persistent wheeze showed a similar distribution. However, there were only small differences in the prevalence of asthma attacks by ethnicity. The large difference in persistent wheeze and the lack of it for asthma attacks between groups suggests that persistent wheeze is unrecognized as asthma in a large percentage of children from the ethnic minorities.

The low frequency of wheeze in children from the Indian subcontinent in comparison to other groups was studied further by assessing the prevalence of exercise-induced BHR (bronchial responsiveness) in 9-year-olds. Children were asked to ride a cycle ergometer for 6 minutes. Their PEFR (peak expiratory flow rate) was measured before exercise and at 5 and 10 minutes after its completion (Jones *et al*. 1996). A 15% or greater decrease of PEFR was defined as positive

Table 9.3 Prevalence of asthma or wheeze and exercise-induced bronchial responsiveness by ethnic group in 9-year-olds

	Number of children	Asthma or wheeze (%)	Bronchial responsiveness (%)
White inner city	155	15.9	4.5
Afro-Caribbean	55	23.7	9.1
Indian subcontinent	138	6.8	12.3
White Scottish representative sample	193	10.9	2.6

Taken from Jones *et al.*, Thorax, 1996, **51**, 1134–36; with permission from the *BMJ* Publishing Group.

Table 9.4 Mean ratio of FVC, FEV_1, and FEF_{25-75} for inner-city and Scottish children to that of the English white representative sample

	Number of children	FVC	FEV_{1-}	FEF_{25-75}
Boys				
White inner city	184	0.99	0.99	1.02
Afro-Caribbean	67	0.84	0.87	1.01
Indian subcontinent	241	0.90	0.91	1.03
Scottish sample	195	1.04	1.04	1.07
Girls				
White inner city	195	0.98	0.99	1.03
Afro-Caribbean	71	0.89	0.90	0.98
Indian subcontinent	179	0.88	0.90	1.01
Scottish sample	173	1.05	1.07	1.14

Taken from Chinn and Rona, *Thorax*, 1992, **47**, 707–14; with permission from *BMJ* Publishing Group.

bronchoconstriction. Children from the Indian subcontinent had the highest prevalence of BHR (12%), followed by Afro-Caribbeans (9%). White children in inner-city areas (4.5%) and Scottish children (3%) had the lowest percentage of BHR (Table 9.3). In this group the percentage of children from the Indian subcontinent with asthma or wheeze was 7%, the lowest in comparison to any other ethnic group. With the exception of the children from the Asian subcontinent there was a correspondence between parental reporting of asthma attacks and/or wheeze and exercise-induced BHR. The low prevalence of asthma symptoms in the Indian subcontinent group, based on parental perception, is also contradicted by the higher percentage of casualty attendance and hospital admissions in this group than among white children (Ayres 1986; Pararajasingam *et al.* 1992). Our results suggest that there is a differential perception of asthmatic symptoms between ethnic groups. Either parents from the Indian subcontinent underreport symptoms of asthma or, less likely, parents from all the other ethnic groups overreport these symptoms.

Using equations adjusted for height and age for the English representative sample, predicted lung function was calculated for the inner-city groups and Scottish sample (Chinn and Rona 1992). The means ratios of actual to predicted values were calculated for each ethnic group for FEV_1, FVC, and FEF_{25-75}. In both sexes Afro-Caribbean and children from the Indian subcontinent had lower values for FVC and FEV_1 than white children from any sample (Table 9.4). Boys from the Afro-Caribbean group had the lowest FVC and FEV_1. Values of FEF_{25-75} were similar between ethnic groups, with the exception of Scottish children, who had higher values than the rest. Low FEV_1 and FVC values in black children have been reported in other studies (Dockery et al. 1983; Patrick and Patel 1986; Schwartz et al. 1988). Schwartz and colleagues (1988) also showed that the differences between black and white children decreased when sitting height was taken into account, but in their study the differences still persisted after adjustment. Thus the differences in lung function between black and white children are due, in part, to differences in body proportion, sitting height being less in relation to total height in blacks than in whites. There are fewer studies comparing the lung function of children from the Indian subcontinent to other ethnic groups, but those available confirm that children from the Indian subcontinent have lower FVC and FEV_1 values than white children (Johnston et al. 1987; Patrick and Patel 1986). It is possible that low lung function in children from the Indian subcontinent, especially in girls, may be due, in part, to the lack of motivation in tests demanding a physical competitive element.

Anthropometric measurements and respiratory illness

Height and respiratory symptoms

There have been many publications assessing the association between height and respiratory illness, especially asthma. However, there is less information on the relation between fatness and respiratory illness. The two issues studied most frequently have been whether children with asthma are shorter than others and whether the use of steroids has an impact on growth in asthmatic children. In the NSHG we have reported the association between respiratory symptoms and height in two papers (Rona and Florey 1980; Somerville and Rona 1993). The first analysis was based on the 1973 survey and the second report was based on the 1984 and 1985 surveys. There were some similarities and differences in the results of the two analyses. Wheeze on most days was negatively associated with height in both surveys after adjustment had been made for a large number of biological and sociodemographic variables. The difference after adjustment was small (1 cm). Occasional wheeze was not associated with height in either survey. Cough during the day or night was highly significantly associated with height, but only in the unadjusted model. The number of asthma attacks was associated with height only in the analysis based on the 1973 survey. Somerville and Rona (1993) carried out an analysis separating children into three groups: those with reported wheeze most days but no asthma attacks; those with wheeze most days and asthma attacks; and those with asthma attacks but not wheeze most days. Wheeze most days but no asthma attacks was negatively associated with height, and wheeze on most days and asthma attacks was only associated with height in the unadjusted model. As in our study, wheeze most days, if not accompanied by a parent's report of asthma attacks in the child, was infrequently treated for asthma, and rarely with steroids at the beginning of the 1990s (Duran-Tauleria et al. 1996), we can assert with confidence that the association of persistent wheeze and height is not related to the use of steroids, and a plausible explanation of our findings is that the severity of asthma symptoms has a small effect on height. This view is further supported by the association of the number of asthma attacks in the analysis based on the 1973 data, but not in the analysis of data from 1984/1985. Duran-Tauleria and colleagues (1996) showed that most children whose parents reported that their child had asthma attacks were treated for asthma. It is probable that by 1984/1985, but not in 1973, children with asthma attacks were prescribed β_2 agonists for the disease, but only a minority were prescribed steroids. Thus the results so far reported can be interpreted as severe asthma affecting height, but we cannot shed any light on the relation between steroids and height in the treatment of asthma. Whether the shorter height of children with persistent wheeze will persist into adulthood is uncertain. Hauspie et al. (1977) showed that asthmatic children are shorter, and also that they had delayed skeletal maturation and their adolescent growth spurt was delayed by 1.3 years. In that study asthmatics reached the height of non-asthmatics as young adults. Whether the characteristics of asthmatic children are now similar to asthmatic children in the 1960s and 1970s is difficult to answer, but if anything children diagnosed as having asthma 30 years ago would have been more severe than nowadays, given the stigma attached to the condition at that time.

In our analysis children with symptoms of cough were not shorter than other children after adjustment for biological and social factors. A possible interpretation of this result is that shorter height and increased cough in these children are characteristics of living in a socially deprived environment.

Respiratory illness and fatness

In an analysis based on data collected in 1977, children with respiratory symptoms and asthma were fatter than other children (Somerville et al. 1984). The analysis was carried out in relation to weight-for-height and triceps skinfold thickness, separately in the English and Scottish samples. In the analysis the dependent variables were respiratory symptoms and the two measures of fatness were independent variables. The percentage of children with colds going to the chest, wheeze, and bronchitis attacks increased as their weight-for-height increased. An undetermined percentage of the children diagnosed as having bronchitis attacks in 1977 would have been classified as having asthma attacks nowadays. The findings of this analysis should be reassessed again using a more recent sample. The association is of interest because the prevalences of both asthma and obesity have greatly increased in Britain over the last 20 years in children and in adults (see Chapters 5 and 11). In adults there are reports of an association between obesity and respiratory illness (Negri et al. 1988; Seidell et al. 1986; Shaheen 1999). In the first of the studies the association was observed only in women (Seidell et al. 1986); in the second it was more related in younger ages than older ages, and the association was J-shaped (Negri et al. 1988). In the recent study the association was seen in both sexes (Shaheen et al. 1999), but it was only statistically significant in women. The evidence so far available on this association is from cross-sectional studies. It is unclear whether those with asthma tend to live a more sedentary lifestyle, obesity is a characteristic that makes more individuals susceptible to asthma, or a combination of the two.

Effects of preterm birth and birthweight on respiratory illness and lung function

Barker (1992) postulated that poor nutrition *in utero* may contribute to the development of several chronic diseases in adulthood. Barker et al. (1992b) showed a negative relation between birthweight and chronic obstructive lung disease mortality and a positive association between birthweight and FEV_1 in adults. Information on the duration of gestation was not collected in their studies. In the NSHG, birthweight and the duration of pregnancy, reported by parents, was available. We also had information on parental smoking. In the analysis a positive association between birthweight and lung function, in terms of FEV_1 and FVC, was found after adjustment for a large number of confounders including gestational age (Rona et al. 1993). Length of gestation was not associated with lung function. However, birthweight was not associated with any of the respiratory symptoms in the study. The main finding in our analysis was that low birthweight and, probably, low intrauterine growth were associated with poor lung growth. This finding is compatible with Barker and colleagues' report in adults.

Length of gestation was associated with wheeze, both persistent and occasional, and cough. Adjustments were made for maternal asthma and birthweight, among other factors, in the analysis.

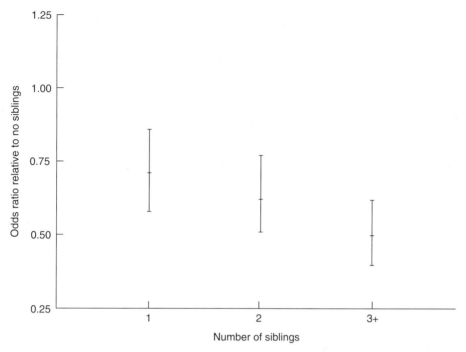

Fig. 9.1   Odds ratio and 95% confidence interval of a child having wheeze or asthma attacks by number of siblings, relative to no sibling in the family. Results taken from Rona *et al.* 1997*a*; with permission.

We concluded that the most plausible interpretation of our results was that fetal immaturity may play a role in the subsequent development of respiratory illness.

Family size, poverty, and asthma

It is generally accepted that there is a predisposition to develop asthma, but that an environmental component also plays an important role in the aetiology of asthma. Using the 1990 and 1991 data we analysed the association between asthma (wheeze or asthma attacks) and family size and birth order, adjusting for atopic conditions in the parents, among other confounding factors (Rona *et al.* 1997*a*). The atopic conditions in the parents for which information was collected were asthma, wheeze, hay fever, rhinitis, and eczema. An association has been shown between birth order and atopic conditions (Strachan 1989; von Mutius *et al.* 1994). Strachan (1997) discussed the hypothesis that repeated viral infections early in life are more frequent in a young child with many older siblings and thus may decrease the chance of a child developing an atopic condition in comparison to an only child. However, there has been little evidence of an association between birth order and asthma (Crane *et al.* 1994). In a logistic regression, in which the dependent variable was dichotomized as children having either asthma attacks or wheeze or neither, we assessed whether family size and, in a separate analysis, birth order were associated with asthma. In the analyses we adjusted for parental atopic conditions, parental smoking, child's gender, ethnicity, father's social class, and geographical area. We showed a very strong association between family size and asthma (Fig. 9.1).

The risk of asthma was doubled in an only child in comparison to children in families with more than three children. The association was not stronger, indeed slightly weaker, when the number of older siblings was entered into the analysis instead of family size. If family size is relevant whatever a child's position in the family, the hypothesis advanced by Strachan (1989) is not entirely satis-factory. An alternative hypothesis, that obesity may be the cause of the association between family size and asthma as an only child in the family tends to have a higher level of fatness than a child with siblings, was also tested. However, adjustment for weight-for-height did not remove the association between asthma and family size. Thus a satisfactory explanation for the association is still unavailable.

We assessed the evolution of the association between family size and asthma in the NSHG covering a 17-year period using data from the 1977, 1985/86, and 1993/94 surveys (Rona et al. 1999). It was puzzling that in the literature the association between asthma and family size was not found in early studies (Davis and Bulpitt 1981; Lewis et al. 1996; Peckham and Butler 1978), while more recent studies have shown the association (Crane et al. 1994; Jarvis et al. 1997; Rona et al. 1997a). In our analysis we showed that there was no association between family size and asthma in the 1977 survey, but in the 1986/87 and 1993/94 surveys families with an only child had more asthma than a child with siblings. The odds ratio was significantly different from 1 only in the 1993/94 data. This second analysis gave limited support to the hypothesis that asthma is currently associated with sibship size. It gave more evidence to show that, if an association does exist, it has arisen only recently. On this evidence the hypothesis that the association between asthma and family size may be due to repeated viral infection is weak.

In our recent analysis (Rona et al. 1999) we also assessed the relation between asthma and father's social class in the three surveys. There has been a change in the association between these two factors. Asthma has become more prevalent in children whose fathers have a manual occupation than in those whose fathers have a non-manual occupation. Within the manual social classes those whose fathers have a semi-skilled or unskilled occupation are at highest risk. The literature on social class and asthma is abundant and contradictory (Mielck et al. 1996). In the 1958 British birth cohort there was no significant association between these two variables (Strachan et al. 1994), but in the 1970 cohort a significant association was found in which 16-year-olds whose fathers were from the managerial social class, or from the semi-skilled and unskilled manual classes, had a higher prevalence of asthma than those from the professional, skilled manual, and non-manual social classes (Lewis et al. 1996).

Mielck and colleagues (1996) hypothesized that severe asthma is associated with social class. The hypothesis is plausible because asthma admission to hospital is high in the poor and ethnic minority groups (Ayres 1986; Carr et al. 1992; Wissow et al. 1988). In community studies some support has been found for this hypothesis (Strachan et al. 1994). In the NSHG we assessed the prevalence of four respiratory symptoms in the 56 study areas: occasional wheeze; persistent wheeze; asthma attacks; and other respiratory symptoms (Duran-Tauleria and Rona, 1999). Persistent wheeze was strongly associated with the father's social class, the Townsend deprivation score of each of the 56 study areas in the study, and ethnic group in the inner-city sample (Fig. 9.2). The Townsend score provides a social deprivation index based on census data on unemployment, car ownership, household overcrowding, and elderly population at postcode sector level (Townsend et al. 1988). The prevalence of persistent wheeze in the inner-city sample was twice that in the English and Scottish representative samples. Adjustment for the Townsend score eliminated the difference in the prevalence of persistent wheeze between the English and each of the groups of the inner-city groups, but adjustment for the father's social class did not eliminate the difference between the two samples. Such heterogeneity by study area was not found for asthma attacks and occasional wheeze, but it was for other respiratory symptoms. Persistent wheeze is the most severe symptom of asthma in our study. Asthma attacks may have indicated severe asthma at the outset of the NSHG,

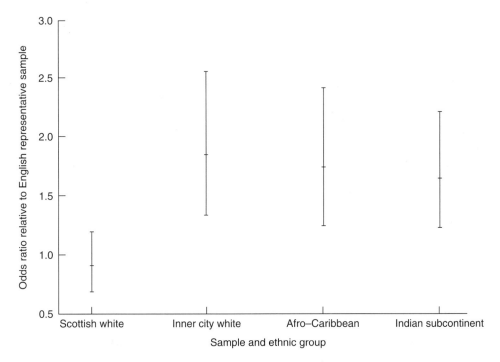

Fig. 9.2   Odds ratio and 95% confidence interval of a child having wheeze or asthma attacks by sample/ethnic origin, relative to English representative sample white children. Results taken from Rona *et al.* 1997*a*; with permission.

but by 1990 children diagnosed as having asthma regardless of severity were ticked positively in the asthma attacks category by their parents. The pattern of the variation of 'other respiratory symptoms' group was similar to persistent wheeze, but the category included a heterogeneous group of symptoms in which an unknown proportion may be children with asthma.

   Our analysis indicated that poverty may be related to severe asthma. The association may be due to lifestyle, material conditions, environmental conditions, or the management of asthma. Of these possibilities we were able to study the management of asthma in the community (Duran-Tauleria *et al.* 1996).

Management of asthma in the community

Underdiagnosis of asthma can lead to undertreatment of the condition, which in turn can cause increased absenteeism from school, attendance at the casualty department, and hospital admission (Gergen and Weiss 1990; Hill *et al.* 1989*a*). Guidelines for the appropriate diagnosis and treatment of asthma have been vigorously disseminated since their publication (Warner *et al.* 1989). In the NSHG, parents were asked to report any drugs taken by the child for respiratory illness in the last 12 months (Duran-Tauleria *et al.* 1996). The drugs were grouped into seven categories: β_2 agonists; other bronchodilators; steroids; other anti-inflammatory drugs; antihistamines; antibiotics; and antitussives. Approximately 82% of children with asthma attacks received a bronchodilator, and a β_2 agonist in 75% of the cases, while only 21% of children with wheeze, either persistent or

Table 9.5   The use of bronchodilators and steroids according to the type of respiratory symptoms

	Number of children	Bronchodilator (%)	Anti-inflammatory drugs	
			Steroids (%)	Other (%)
Asthma attacks	1028	82.5	25.2	14.4
Persistent wheeze but no asthma attacks	404	21.5	4.2	1.2
Occasional wheeze but no asthma attacks	924	21.1	3.6	3.0
Any other respiratory symptom	3138	2.4	0.2	0.3

Duran-Tauleria *et al.* The results were first published in the *BMJ* (Influence of ethnic group on asthma treatment in children in 1990–1; national cross sectional study. *British Medical Journal*, 1996, **313**, 148–52) and are reproduced by permission of the *BMJ*.

occasional, received a bronchodilator if their parents did not report asthma attacks in their child. Approximately 25% of the children with asthma attacks were prescribed steroids and 14% were receiving other anti-inflammatory agents (Table 9.5). Very few children were receiving any anti-inflammatory medicaments among those with persistent or occasional wheeze, but no asthma attacks. It is clear from our analysis that a child reported as having asthma attacks had a high chance of receiving appropriate medication, but those with symptoms of wheeze but not asthma attacks did not. Inappropriate management of the condition was prevalent among children with asthmatic symptoms. Antibiotics were prescribed for approximately 20% of these children regardless of symptoms, and antitussives were prescribed in 11% of children with persistent wheeze despite the lack of evidence of their effectiveness.

Management of asthma was particularly poor among children in the inner-city sample regardless of ethnicity. The chance of a child with any symptom of asthma being prescribed β_2 agonists was less than half in comparison to a child in the English representative sample. The use of β_2 agonists was particularly low in children from the Indian subcontinent. Thus children in the inner-city areas are less likely to be diagnosed as asthmatic and this is likely to lead to poor management of the condition. Although the problem is widespread in inner-city areas it is particularly acute for children of Indian subcontinent origin.

Conclusions

The NSHG has made a sizeable contribution to the understanding of public health issues related to respiratory illness in the community. One of the most important contributions has been to document a series of problems in the management of asthma in inner-city areas and ethnic minorities. The situation of the children of Indian subcontinent origin is illustrative. Our results have shown a mismatch between the relatively low prevalence of asthma symptoms and the high prevalence of exercise-induced bronchial responsiveness in comparisons to other groups. It is possible, therefore, that the recognition of asthmatic symptoms in children from the Indian subcontinent is poor. The problem is compounded by the poor labelling of asthma in all groups in inner-city areas and the poor management of the condition among those diagnosed as having the condition. These characteristics may explain why hospital admissions for asthma are high in poor sectors of the population.

10 Assessing the effect of parental smoking on a child's health

Introduction

When the NSHG was designed the consequences of active smoking had only recently been established, and the notion that passive smoking might also be harmful was in its infancy. Although the data collected on respiratory symptoms were expanded in 1973 (see Table 2.5) information on smoking by parents was not requested until 1977, and did not form part of the core questionnaire until 1987. The literature on the effects of passive smoking is now vast. We consider the contribution of the NSHG to the accumulated evidence in relation to three outcomes: growth; lung function; and respiratory symptoms.

Growth

An observation in another study prompted an analysis of a child's height in relation to the number of smokers in the home using the 1977 data (Rona *et al*. 1981). A negative relation between a child's height and the number of smokers was found, but the relation was reduced on adjustment for confounding factors, particularly the number of siblings. As described in Chapter 6, the number of siblings has been found to be consistently associated with a child's height in the representative samples, independently of other factors. Adequate adjustment for potentially confounding factors is essential in an observational study, particularly when the effect to be estimated is likely to be small in relation to the major determinants of outcome. In the analysis of the 1977 data the relation remained after adjusting for birthweight, leading the authors to conclude that the known adverse effect of maternal smoking in pregnancy on birthweight was not responsible for the relation between height and smoking in the home.

In 1982 questions on parental smoking were included in order to re-examine the issue. Data on the number of cigarettes smoked in total and at home, for each parent, were collected, and on whether the mother smoked when she was pregnant with the child. In a multiple regression analysis the relation of height to the total number of cigarettes smoked daily in the home remained negative and statistically significant after adjustment for mother smoking in pregnancy, parental heights, birthweight, number of older siblings, social class, and several other variables (Rona *et al*. 1985).

Data on smoking were not collected again until 1987, due to caution over the length of the core questionnaire when the inner-city sample was first recruited in 1983, and the need for dual language questionnaires (Chapter 3). Data from both representative samples and the inner-city sample were included in an analysis of the 1987 and 1988 data (Chinn and Rona 1991). In this analysis the total number of siblings was included as a categorical variable, whereas in the earlier analysis it was assumed that the trend in height with the number of older siblings was linear. No significant relation of height to the number of cigarettes smoked at home by the parents was found in any ethnic group. The overall regression coefficient of height SDS on the daily number of cigarettes was 0.0003 (95% confidence interval, −0.0016 to 0.0022). When the 1982 data were reanalysed correspondingly the size of effect was reduced, and no longer statistically significant. It was concluded that the relation of height to passive smoking was not substantiated. However, the earlier paper has been referenced in relation to growth in an extensive review of the effects of passive smoking on children (Charlton 1994), despite the later paper being cited elsewhere in the same review. In a longitudinal study in the United States Berkey et al. (1984) found a relation between attained height of 6–11-year-old children and the number of cigarettes smoked by the mother, but no relation with rate of growth. They concluded that these results were evidence that the relation of attained height to passive smoking was due to exposure *in utero* or during infancy, and that continuing exposure was unlikely to have any further effect.

Lung function

A number of studies, mainly in the United States, had looked at the relation of lung function to passive smoking prior to spirometry being performed in the NSHG for children aged 7–11 years from 1987 to 1990. The only British studies were small in comparison. Although most of the American studies found some relation the results were not entirely consistent, in particular between the two longitudinal studies. Using comparable analyses the East Boston study found a relation between FEV_1 and maternal smoking, but the Tucson study did not (Lebowitz and Holberg 1988; Tager et al. 1987). One large cross-sectional study (Ware et al. 1984), of nearly 9000 children aged between 6 and 9 years at the first examination, reported lower FEV_1 but greater FVC in children of parents who both smoked compared to that of children of non-smoking parents. Mid-expiratory flow rates were not analysed. The largest study (Hasselblad et al. 1981), of 16 689 children aged from 6 to 13 years, found a relation of $FEV_{0.75}$ to the amount smoked by the mother, but no relation to parental smoking. The other studies included older children in whom active smoking may be difficult to exclude, and the East Boston study looked at the relation only to maternal smoking in the later papers (Tager et al. 1983, 1987). The method of adjustment for height and age also varied between studies, and the number of smokers in the home rather than the amount smoked was used to examine a dose–response relation.

The NSHG data provided an opportunity to estimate the relation of lung function to the number of cigarettes smoked in the home, by father and mother separately and in total, in an age group in which active smoking was unlikely to confound the relation. The methodology for the adjustment of lung function for height and age, described in Chapter 2, was developed before any analysis in relation to passive smoking was attempted. Although some evidence of a negative relation of FEF_{25-75} and FEF_{75-85} to maternal smoking was found in 1429 boys (Rona and Chinn 1993), it was weaker in the 1309 girls, and with just 2 out of 16 analyses giving statistically significant results the findings might have arisen by chance. On the other hand, the results did not preclude small associations such as those found by Hasselblad et al. (1981).

Since 1993 more studies have been published, and further follow-up reported from the American longitudinal studies. D. G. Cook et al. (1998) identified 42 population-based studies that reported on the cross-sectional relation between some measure of parental smoking and spirometric indices in children. Using meta-analysis methods they combined the results from 22 studies to provide estimates of the effect of parental smoking on FVC, FEV_1, mid-expiratory flow, and end-expiratory flow, expressed as a percentage difference between the exposed and non-exposed groups. However, they were forced to combine the estimates from studies that looked at maternal smoking only, those that compared either parent smoking with neither, those that compared both parents smoking with neither, and those that contrasted the top quintile of urinary cotinine level with the lowest quintile. FEF_{25-75} was assumed to be equivalent to FEF_{50}, and FEF_{75} to FEF_{85}. Despite this no study had data for all four indices, the maximum being 21 for FEV, decreasing to just nine for end-expiratory flow. Data for boys and girls separately were available from just nine studies. The authors commented that it was not surprising that heterogeneity between the studies was detected.

Given these problems it is difficult to understand why the NSHG results were not included in the meta-analysis, although the study was among the 42 identified and was one of the larger studies. The reason given was that the NSHG 'reported differences in standard deviation scores with no baseline data'. However, as the standard deviation scores (SDS) were calculated using the mean and standard deviation of the ratio of actual to predicted lung function for height, age, and gender (Chinn and Rona 1992) the SDS can be converted to the ratio scale by multiplying by the appropriate standard deviation. These were published (Chinn and Rona 1992), and the results of Rona and Chinn (1993) have been converted to the percentage effect of two parents smoking 20 cigarettes a day in the home or one parent smoking 10 (Table 10.1). These figures are likely to be an overestimate of the average number smoked in the home (Chinn and Rona 1991), but nevertheless the estimates in Table 10.1 are either positive, or less negative, than the estimates of D. G. Cook *et al.* (1998). Our results are not in conflict with the meta-analysis results, as the confidence intervals in Table 10.1 are wide enough to include the small but statistically significant reductions in FEV_1, mid-expiratory flow and end-expiratory flow, and the non-significant result for FVC found by D. G. Cook *et al.* (1998). Inclusion of the NSHG results in the meta-analysis would have decreased the size of the estimated reductions in lung function.

D. G. Cook *et al.* (1998) did reference the NSHG results in commenting that 'of 10 studies which allow comparison of the effects of maternal and paternal smoking nearly all report the effect of maternal smoking to be greater than that of paternal smoking'. Our results also support the finding that the passive smoking effect was larger for mid- and end-expiratory flow rates than for FEV_1, although the confidence intervals are also wider. Like the majority of studies that analysed the effect separately for boys and girls (D. G. Cook *et al.* 1998), we commented that the effects were greater in boys than in girls, but the difference was not statistically significant. D. G. Cook *et al.* combined the gender difference across nine studies not including the NSHG results, obtaining a *p*-value of 0.06.

Although the longitudinal data are now extensive the question of whether the cross-sectional relation of lung function to passive smoking is due entirely to lasting effects of prenatal and postnatal exposure, or in part to current exposure remains unanswered. D. G. Cook *et al.* (1998) were clearly disappointed to find that none of the longitudinal studies had looked at change in lung function in relation to change in exposure. Chinn (1989*b*) had discussed the need for such an analysis, but as D. G. Cook *et al.* point out such a study would require good estimates of exposure. Until such a study is carried out the question will remain unanswered.

Respiratory symptoms

The data on passive smoking were collected in 1977 for an analysis of the relation of respiratory illness to the use of gas for cooking in the home (Melia *et al.* 1979). Passive smoking was a potential confounding variable, and not studied in detail. As described above the first full analysis was in relation to growth, not respiratory symptoms. By the mid-1980s a number of studies had been published; but while these were consistent in suggesting increased infections in children under 1 year of age exposed to parental smoking, a review article (Guyatt and Newhouse 1985) concluded that studies in older children were inconsistent.

The 1982 data were analysed taking a number of confounding variables into account. The prevalence of wheeze, attacks of bronchitis in the last 12 months, day or night cough, and at least one of six respiratory conditions showed significant relations to the number of cigarettes smoked by parents in the home in over 4300 English children with complete data, and for wheeze and the

Table 10.1 The percentage difference in spirometric indices associated with total parental smoking of 20 cigarettes a day at home, or of 10 cigarettes a day by one parent at home

Exposure	Sample size	FVC (95% CI) (%)	FEV_1 (95% CI) (%)	FEF_{25-75} (95% CI) (%)	FEF_{75-85} (95% CI) (%)
Boys					
20 cigarettes a day at home	1429	0.26 (−0.97 to 1.50)	−0.47 (−1.75 to 0.81)	−2.57 (−5.33 to 0.19)*	−3.49 (−7.99 to 1.02)
10 cigarettes a day by mother	1470	−0.17 (−1.11 to 0.76)	−0.84 (−1.78 to 0.12)	−3.11 (−5.15 to −1.06)***	−3.96 (−6.29 to −1.63)**
10 cigarettes a day by father	1388	0.45 (−0.52 to 1.44)	0.42 (−0.59 to 1.45)	0.36 (−1.82 to 2.55)	1.27 (−2.38 to 4.92)
Girls					
20 cigarettes a day at home	1309	0.35 (−0.97 to 1.67)	−0.25 (−1.71 to 1.21)	−2.46 (−5.55 to 0.62)	−0.85 (−5.42 to 3.71)
10 cigarettes a day by mother	1342	−0.15 (−1.15 to 0.85)	−0.58 (−1.68 to 0.51)	−1.44 (−3.75 to 0.87)	−1.13 (−4.63 to 2.37)
10 cigarettes a day by father	1273	0.82 (−0.20 to 1.85)	0.72 (−0.40 to 1.84)	−0.52 (−2.94 to 1.89)	1.32 (−2.26 to 4.90)

CI confidence interval: *$p < 0.1$; **$p < 0.05$; ***$p < 0.01$.
Derived from Rona and Chinn 1993.

Table 10.2 Odds ratios for respiratory conditions associated with 20 cigarettes smoked by parents in the home, estimated by weighted average of results for white boys and girls in English and Scottish representative samples and English inner-city sample

Respiratory condition	Odds ratio (95% confidence interval)
Chest EVER wheezy or whistling	1.13 (1.00 to 1.27)
Chest wheezy or whistling on MOST days or nights	1.38 (1.25 to 1.52)
In last 12 months	
Bronchitis	1.08 (0.87 to 1.25)
Asthma	1.02 (0.92 to 1.13)
Usually coughs	1.30 (1.22 to 1.38)
At least one condition	1.17 (1.11 to 1.25)

Derived from Chinn and Rona 1991.

prevalence of at least one condition in over 750 Scottish children (Somerville *et al.* 1988). The results were compatible with previous large studies that also had data to study a dose–response relation in a similar age group.

As described above for growth, a reanalysis was possible following the collection of further data in 1987 and 1988. As these data were designed to test the hypothesis of a relation of respiratory symptoms to passive smoking, unlike the 1982 data, information on the use of a gas cooker or paraffin heater in the home was also collected. In addition to these two variables the relation of respiratory symptoms to the number of cigarettes smoked per day at home was adjusted for the child's age, ethnic origin, and birthweight as well as the number of siblings, father's social class, home overcrowding, maternal age, whether part of a one-parent family, mother's education, whether the mother smoked in pregnancy with the child, and whether in receipt of free school meals. Results combined across the three samples, for boys and girls, and adapted from the published paper (Chinn and Rona 1991), are summarized in Table 10.2. The trends were positive for all respiratory conditions, and statistically significant for wheeze on most days or nights ($p < 0.01$), usual cough ($p < 0.001$), and at least one condition ($p < 0.01$).

It was clear that no one study would convince the scientific community that there was a relation between parental smoking and respiratory symptoms in children. The literature is now extensive, and as part of a series on the health effects of passive smoking D. G. Cook and Strachan (1997) have reviewed the evidence in school-age children. They identified 60 studies providing quantitative estimates of the relation of symptoms and asthma to either parent smoking, which were combined in a random effects meta-analysis. They found odds ratios greater than one, with strong evidence against no effect, for asthma, wheeze, cough, phlegm, and breathlessness. They concluded that the relation of respiratory symptoms to parental smoking was very likely to be causal, given the statistical significance, robustness to adjustment for confounding variables, and the consistency of findings in different studies. As the studies were cross-sectional the age at which the adverse effects occurred could not be determined, but D. G. Cook and Strachan (1997) argued that the raised risk in households where the father, but not the mother, smoked, was evidence for a postnatal effect.

The two NSHG studies (Chinn and Rona 1991; Somerville *et al.* 1988) contributed to the estimates for asthma, wheeze, and chronic cough, and the later study was one of the largest identified. Each study also adjusted for more variables than the majority of the other studies, some of which provided no adjustment for confounding. For asthma, the NSHG provided 2 out of 10 adjusted estimates, for wheeze 2 out of 14, and for cough 2 out of 12. Hence, although the meta-analysis could have been conducted without the NSHG results it is clear that they made a substantial contribution to the review. In addition, the NSHG has provided estimates of the dose–response effect, whereas the majority of studies had data only on whether the parents smoked.

Conclusions

Of the three aspects of passive smoking in children that have been studied using NSHG data, the contribution in relation to respiratory symptoms has been greatest. We were a little surprised to demonstrate a relation of symptoms to passive smoking in the 1982 data, but the subsequent confirmation using the 1987 and 1988 data removed our scepticism. We believe that the review by D. G. Cook and Strachan (1997) should be the last word on the subject of the cross-sectional relation of symptoms to passive smoking, although the NSHG is one of the few studies to provide estimates of the size of the effects. The same is true of the relation of lung function to passive smoking, and it is disappointing to find that our careful methodological work on the appropriate analysis of lung function in children led to our results not being included in the meta-analysis of D. G. Cook et al. (1998). The early report of a relation to height, which was later retracted, nevertheless continues to be quoted, illustrating the need to retain objectivity over an issue that is emotive.

11 Secular trend in asthma

Background

The first studies to indicate a rise in the prevalence of asthma in schoolchildren came from Birmingham where schoolchildren were studied in 1956/7, 1968/9, and 1974/5. The prevalence of asthma or wheeze rose substantially in the first period and continued to rise, although at a lower rate in the second period of study (Morrison Smith 1976). Interpretation of the increase was, however, difficult as Birmingham was being rebuilt at this time and there were considerable changes in the population. Confirmation of this increase in asthma prevalence in Britain was provided by a study conducted in Caerphilly, Wales (Burr et al. 1989), but, although this study was situated in a town with a more stable population, it was based on only two points in time. Several British authors pointed to the lack of a trend in estimates of wheezing illness over time (Anderson 1989b; Hay and Higginbottam 1987), and a further study over a very short time period failed to show a significant increase in wheezing (Hill et al. 1989b). An analysis based on data collected between 1973 and 1986 in the English areas of the NSHG was able to provide strong support for the view that the increase in the prevalence of asthma was real, was geographically widespread, and continued over a substantial period of time (Burney et al. 1990).

First report

Information on wheeze, both persistent or occasional, was collected in most surveys, except between 1978 and 1981; information on asthma or bronchitis in the previous 12 months was available from the follow-up questionnaire administered from 1973 to 1976, and for all children from then on. The information was divided by gender and into cohort by year of birth. Table 11.1

Table 11.1   Trends in the prevalence of asthma and asthma symptoms from 1973 to 1986 (England)

Symptom or condition	Trend in prevalence per annual cohort (%)	
	Boys	Girls
Asthma	6.9[**]	12.8[**]
Bronchitis	−4.7[**]	−5.5[**]
Occasional wheeze	1.0	1.7
Persistent wheeze	4.3[**]	6.1[**]
Asthma or bronchitis	−1.6[*]	−0.1
Persistent wheeze, no asthma or bronchitis	11.1[**]	4.5[*]

$^*p < 0.05$; $^{**}p < 0.01$.

Burney et al. The results were first published in the BMJ (Has the prevalence of asthma increased in children? Evidence from the national study of health and growth 1973–86. British Medical Journal, 1990, **300**, 1306–10) and are reproduced by permission of the BMJ.

Table 11.2 Age-adjusted odds ratios for respiratory symptoms and conditions in 1992 compared to 1982 in English and Scottish boys and girls

Symptom or condition	England		Scotland	
	Boys	Girls	Boys	Girls
Asthma attacks	3.0***	2.7***	2.8***	3.0***
Bronchitis attacks	0.7	0.7	0.3***	0.5**
Occasional wheeze	1.6***	1.5***	1.3**	1.3*
Persistent wheeze	1.4*	1.4*	1.1	1.2
Persistent wheeze, no asthma or bronchitis	0.9	1.5	0.9	0.8

$^*p < 0.05$; $^{**}p < 0.01$; $^{***}p < 0.001$ (difference from 1.0).
Taken from Rona et al., Thorax, 1995, **50**, 992–3; with permission from the BMJ Publishing Group.

shows the estimated trends within age group per annual cohort for asthma, bronchitis, and wheeze. There was a substantial increase in asthma and a substantial decrease in bronchitis in both sexes. This can be construed as an increasing awareness of asthma rather than a genuine increase in the prevalence of the condition. It is well known that correct labelling is associated with specific management of the condition (Duran-Tauleria et al. 1996; Speight et al. 1983) and there had been considerable pressure on doctors from the early 1980s onwards to make the diagnosis and prescribe adequate treatment. However, a large increase in persistent wheeze in boys and girls was also found. This trend was observed both in children with persistent wheeze only and in children reported to have attacks of asthma or bronchitis. This indicates that the increase in prevalence was not due solely to changes in medical practice. In this analysis, milder forms of wheeze did not increase to the same extent as persistent wheeze. Thus either more severe forms of the condition increased or the population became slightly more prone to wheeze, with a consequent greater proportional increase in the prevalence of severe disease. Occasional wheeze may be subject to higher rates of misclassification. Burr and colleagues (1989) found a greater increase in exercise-induced bronchial responsiveness at the severe end of the distribution.

The strength of the evidence from the NSHG arises from the multiple measurements of symptoms over a substantial period of time in a large number of areas. These give a much greater certainty that what is being observed is a trend rather than just a difference between two points in time, and that the result is not unduly affected by demographic changes in a particular area as may have occurred in Birmingham. It was also possible in this study to distinguish diagnoses from symptoms and to analyse these separately.

Replication of the findings

The trend in the prevalence of asthma was assessed again, using the same respiratory symptoms and conditions, in England and Scotland for the period between 1982/83 and 1992/93 (Rona et al. 1995). As described in Chapter 2 from 1982/83 the number of study areas in Scotland was increased to 14, which allowed us to carry out a worthwhile analysis on the Scottish sample. The English representative sample was also included in the analysis to ascertain whether a further increase had occurred since the first analysis and also for comparison with the Scottish sample. Table 11.2 shows the odds ratios (OR) of respiratory symptoms by gender and country. In the two samples the OR for asthma markedly increased over the period. Occasional wheeze also increased over the period in both countries. Persistent wheeze also increased significantly ($p < 0.05$) in England, but not in Scotland. The continuing large increase in asthma and decrease in bronchitis indicated that diagnostic behaviour continued to change over this period. However, the increase in persistent wheeze in England supports the view that at least part of this increase was real. In Scotland, the lack of a significant increase of persistent wheeze over the period may have been due to the unusually high prevalence for this symptom in Scotland in the 1982/83 surveys in comparison to the subsequent 1984/85 surveys. By the time this paper was published there was additional evidence in support of a real increase in asthma prevalence in Scotland (Ninan and Russell 1992), though based on two surveys using different methodology, and England (Anderson *et al*. 1994), but the increase in the latter study was small. By this time there was evidence for an increase in asthma prevalence from 11 different countries (Burney 1997).

Apart from the widespread replication of these findings there were two other pieces of evidence that suggested that the increase was real. These two studies of schoolchildren had shown an increase in bronchial responsiveness that coincided with an increase in symptoms (Burr *et al*. 1989; Peat *et al*. 1994), and a number of studies had shown increases in the prevalence of other atopic diseases at the same time (Burr *et al*. 1989; Ninan and Russell 1992).

In addition to the studies that have collected information on both asthma and other allergic conditions there have been independent reports of increases in the prevalence of eczema (Schultz Larsen *et al*. 1986; Taylor *et al*. 1984), although there is much less information on hay fever. Nevertheless, there is also evidence that the prevalence of specific IgE to common aeroallergens has also increased in schoolchildren (Gassner 1992; Nakagomi *et al*. 1994). This provides support for an increase in skin sensitivity over time based on a methodology that is more difficult to standardize. Even though this evidence suggests that an increase in sensitization may explain some of the increase in asthma it is likely that this is not the whole explanation. The increases in symptoms and hyperresponsiveness reported from New South Wales were not accompanied by an increase in atopy as measured by skin tests (Peat *et al*. 1994) and, although this may be explained by the difficulty of standardizing skin tests, it is a finding that appears to agree with other data from Australia.

Several explanations have been suggested for the increase in the prevalence of atopy or asthma over time, including increasing allergen exposure, smoking, family size, diet, and obesity. Although there is evidence that 'tight housing' may increase an exposure to allergens (Luczynska *et al*. 1990), there is little direct evidence that exposure to allergens has increased over the past decades. Sporik *et al*. (1990) were unable to show an increase in house dust-mite allergens in homes in one study in southern England between 1979/80 and 1989. The length and intensity of the grass pollen season have reduced, if anything (Emberlin *et al*. 1993) and Seaton and colleagues (1994) have argued from trends in the sales of pet food that there is little evidence for an increase in pet keeping.

The effects of smoking and passive smoking are complex. Magnusson (1986) reported an increased concentration of IgE in the cord blood of children from mothers who smoke during pregnancy. However, the finding has not been replicated. In adults, smoking is associated with an increased incidence of sensitization to occupational allergens (Zetterstrom *et al*. 1981), and possibly to dust-mite allergens, but not to other common aeroallergens (Jarvis *et al*. 1995; Omenaas *et al*. 1994). It has been known for a long time that the children of mothers who smoke have more respiratory disease in infancy (Colley *et al*. 1974) and, though this association weakens over time (Fergusson *et al*. 1981), it is still detectable in studies at later years. Asthma is associated with parental smoking (Chapter 10). The trend in women's smoking does not fit well with the trends in childhood asthma.

Many authors have now shown a link between atopic conditions and small sibships (Lebowitz *et al*. 1987; Strachan 1989), though it has been much less common to find any association between sibship size and asthma. This issue has already been addressed in Chapter 9. Again, there is very little evidence that family size has changed over recent decades in such a way as to explain trends in asthma prevalence (OPCS 1987).

Some commentators have suggested that changes in diet may have been responsible for the increase in asthma (Seaton *et al.* 1994). However, there are still inadequate data to implicate any particular dietary constituent in asthma prevalence (Weiss 1997), let alone for the increasing prevalence of asthma. There is, however, emerging evidence of an association between obesity and asthma (Kaplan and Montana 1993; Luder *et al.* 1998; Somerville *et al.* 1984). The direction of causality between the two variables is unclear. As described in Chapter 5, obesity has also increased over the period of the study. There is insufficient information to fully support the hypothesis, but it seems reasonable to explore it further.

Conclusions

Parental perception of asthma symptoms in the NSHG has been helpful in documenting an increase in asthma and wheezy illness in children over the period of the study. Unlike the majority of studies the NSHG provided data at more than two time points and with a geographical spread of the study population. We have documented an increase in asthma that could be related to changes in perception, recognition, and labelling. However, the increase in persistent wheeze, which may be independent of labelling, is strong evidence that there has been a real increase in the prevalence of asthma. There are several competing explanations for the phenomenon, but the evidence so far available is insufficient for supporting one of them unequivocally.

12 Parents' perceptions of their child's health

Background

The NSHG allowed us to explore the magnitude of health and social issues in childhood as perceived by parents. Among several subjects we studied food intolerance, disturbed sleep, and nocturnal enuresis. In the case of food intolerance our interest was to assess whether its public perception as a widespread health problem and the media attention received translated to parents' perceptions of food intolerance in children. In parallel with this public perception of the problem there was also an increasing realization that health professionals were inconsistent in their response to consultations about the problem. Our interest in sleep was restricted at the outset to assessing the association between duration of sleep at night and height in children. It is well known that growth hormone levels increase during sleep (Hunter and Rigal 1966; Takahashi et al. 1968) and we wanted to assess whether children whose parents reported their child sleeping long hours tended to be taller than other children. We did not find a positive association between sleep duration and growth, if anything the opposite was shown (Gulliford et al. 1990). Subsequently we became interested in exploring disturbed sleep as the epidemiological literature was scant. In these studies it was not feasible to refine the diagnosis based on parents' views. However, whether or not the child had a clinical condition, parents' perceptions had an effect on the functioning of the family and its demand for health services. Nocturnal enuresis was included in the questionnaire because it was considered that disturbed sleep should be analysed in the context of whether or not it was accompanied by other symptoms or conditions.

Parents' perceptions of food intolerance

Food intolerance is a term used to describe an abnormal physiological response to an ingested food or food additive (Sampson 1997). Sampson excluded food allergy from the definition of food intolerance, but in the NSHG the term was used to be inclusive of any reaction to food regardless of the mechanism. It included idiosyncratic responses to food, and allergy to food and food additives. Although in some cases the reaction to food consumption follows within a few minutes and the association is fairly clear, the relation between the two events is unclear in the majority of the cases. Double-blind, placebo-controlled food challenge is considered the standard criterion for diagnosis, but again it is not easy to distinguish cases of food intolerance in community studies (Young et al. 1987, 1994). Delayed reactions, the amount eaten, an interaction of the offending food with other intervening factors, e.g. exercise, and the contribution of emotional problems make the diagnosis of food intolerance difficult.

In 1984 we assessed the prevalence of the condition as perceived by parents, its distribution in the community, and its associations with illness. We also asked about the type of food identified as causing the reaction. As height is considered a good measure of nutritional status we assessed whether there was a difference in height between children with food intolerance and those who were not considered intolerant by their parents. The questions asked were 'Has this child ever had an

Table 12.1   Child's prevalence of symptoms according to parent's perception of food intolerance

Condition	Intolerant No. (%)	Uncertain No. (%)	Tolerant No. (%)
Eczema	177 (33)	101 (14)	6348 (6)
Hives	170 (11)	99 (9)	6291 (2)
Hay fever	172 (21)	99 (14)	6321 (6)
Asthma	191 (19)	105 (10)	6475 (4)
Wheeze	189 (36)	104 (18)	6521 (10)
Headache	174 (13)	96 (13)	6268 (2)
Rhinitis	172 (22)	98 (21)	6310 (6)
Diarrhoea and vomiting	168 (12)	99 (5)	6287 (1)
Irritability	170 (17)	97 (6)	6271 (2)

Rona and Chinn. The results were first published in the *BMJ* (Parents' perceptions of food intolerance in primary school children. *British Medical Journal*, 1987*b*, **294**, 863–6) and are reproduced by permission of the *BMJ*.

Table 12.2   Prevalence of food intolerance and maternal level of education

Mother's level of education	Child food status			
	Intolerant (%)	Uncertain (%)	Tolerant (%)	Total no. (%)
No formal education	0	2	98	55
Primary education	1	0	99	195
Secondary school	2	1	97	4311
Commercial or technical	4	2	94	1276
University	6	5	90	344

Rona and Chinn. The results were first published in the *BMJ* (Parents' perceptions of food intolerance in primary school children. *British Medical Journal*, 1987*b*, **294**, 863–6) and are reproduced by permission of the *BMJ*.

illness or trouble caused by eating a particular food or foods?' and 'Has this child nearly always had the same illness or trouble after eating this type of food?'. We defined as food intolerant those whose parent replied affirmatively to both questions, and as uncertain those for whom the reply was positive only to the first question (Rona and Chinn 1987*b*). Of the total, 2.8% of the children were considered food intolerant and 1.4% uncertain whether food intolerant. The food items most likely to be avoided were orange squash, milk, eggs, oranges or lemons, chocolate, fish or shellfish, nuts, fish fingers, and flour. Of the children classified as food intolerant 90% were avoiding at least one type of food. The type and frequency of food items avoided were similar regardless of whether the decision to eliminate the food item came from health staff or the parents themselves. Approximately 9% of the children in the not food intolerant group were also avoiding a food item for health reasons. The ranking of food avoided was different in the two groups. In the food intolerant group the food eliminated matched the list of food usually quoted as causing food intolerance in the scientific literature, while in the tolerant group some of the items avoided may have been eliminated from the diet for other reasons, for example the child's fads. Each of the symptoms explored was more frequent in food intolerant children than other children (Table 12.1). Even a child's irritability as assessed by parents or others was associated with food intolerance after allowing for other diseases such as eczema and asthma (Price *et al.* 1990).

Food intolerance was highly associated with the mother's educational level (Table 12.2). There are many explanations for the high prevalence of food intolerance in children of mothers with a

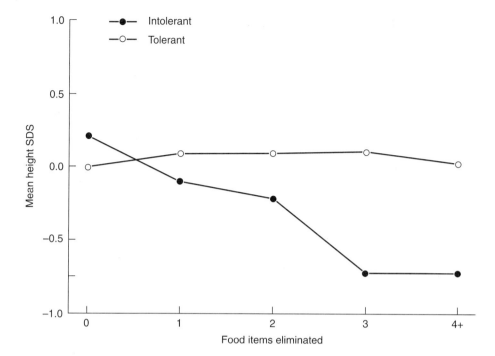

Fig. 12.1   Mean height (SDS) of food intolerant and non-food intolerant children by the number of food items eliminated from the diet. Results taken from Price *et al.* (Height of primary school children and parents' perceptions of food intolerance. *British Medical Journal*, 1988, **296**, 1696–9) and are reproduced by permission of the *BMJ*.

university education. They may be more perceptive of issues related to food than other mothers, they may be more influenced by the media, or the conditions associated with food intolerance may be more prevalent in higher social classes.

Food intolerant children were shorter by 0.3 SDS (approximately 2 cm) than children who were not food intolerant. After adjustment for social factors and biological factors usually highly associated with height in children (see Chapter 6) the difference in height remained between the groups. The height difference was equivalent to that associated with a difference of 1 kg in birthweight or a difference in maternal height of 6 cm. However, the percentage of children with height two SDS below the mean was only slightly higher (4%) than expected in the total population (2.3%) and not statistically significant. We found an association between the number of food items eliminated from the diet and height in the food intolerant group, but not in the food tolerant (Fig 12.1). Children who had three or more food items eliminated from the diet were substantially shorter than children for whom less than two items were eliminated, in the food intolerant group (3 to 4 cm). The mean values were adjusted for social and biological factors usually found associated with height in the NSHG (Chapter 6).

A possible explanation for our results is that concurrent conditions or symptoms reported by the parents may have caused height deterioration in these children. We tested this possibility by adjusting for the conditions explored in the study and found that the differences in height remained almost unchanged (Price *et al.* 1988). The most likely explanations for our finding are that either the number of food items eliminated from the diet is a reflection of the severity of the underlying condition or that the foods eliminated from the diet were not replaced appropriately in terms of nutrients. It is known that decreased growth is a common problem in children with a well-characterized food intolerance, but most of the reports refer to coeliac disease or allergy to cows' milk (Groll *et al.* 1980; Stern and Walker 1985). Two recent reviews have reported that it is rare for a food intolerant child to be intolerant to more than one food item (Chandra 1997; Sampson 1997). Therefore the most likely reason for avoiding several food items for a long period of time without continuous assessment is that health staff or parents are unable to identify the food item causing the symptoms. In our study only 26% of those classified as food intolerant did not consult a doctor. Although substantial, this percentage is small in comparison to the percentage not consulting for other conditions studied in the NSHG, such as disturbed sleep and enuresis. The conclusions from 10 years ago are still appropriate: first, that specialists and general practitioners should define clear criteria for the diagnosis and management of food intolerance; and second, when parents complain of food intolerance in a child the complaint needs to be taken seriously by health staff, as the child may suffer, either from the condition or as a consequence of the management of an unsubstantiated condition.

Disturbed sleep and enuresis

Sleep disorders in children are classified into two major groups: the dyssomnias, difficulty in initiating or maintaining sleep; and parasomnias, disorders that disrupt sleep after it has been initiated (Adair and Bauchner 1993). Nocturnal enuresis (referred to as enuresis from now on) has been included in the second group. The epidemiological literature on enuresis is considerable and has a long history, but studies on disturbed sleep are scarce and most include only preschool children. From this perspective it is appropriate to discuss enuresis as a separate entity from disturbed sleep. A common feature of both conditions is that they may create distress in the child and the family. Chronic fatigue in parents, curtailment of social and family life, and parental violence are common phenomena accompanying these disorders (Kerr and Jowett 1994; Warzak 1993).

Enuresis

Enuresis has been seen as a condition that is strongly environmentally determined (Blomfield and Douglas 1956; Essen and Peckham 1976; Golding and Tissier 1986; Miller *et al.* 1974). Although rarely studied, a familial component has also been acknowledged (Bakwin 1971). Figure 12.2 shows the prevalence of frequent enuresis (i.e. at least once a week) by age and gender. Enuresis is more frequent in boys than girls and decreases sharply with age, but even in 11-year-old girls the frequency is approximately 2%. Enuresis is more frequent in Afro-Caribbean children, in children with older siblings, in those whose mother smokes, and in children of younger mothers (Table 12.3). In our analysis there was an association between the father's social class and enuresis, but only in girls. This was also reported by Blomfield and Douglas (1956). When comparing studies over the last 45 years it is interesting that the prevalence of enuresis has not decreased despite changes in the social and material environment in Britain (Rona *et al.* 1997b). This indicates that material conditions are less likely to influence enuresis than cultural characteristics of deprivation. This is compatible with the association of enuresis with younger mothers, maternal smoking, family size, and, perhaps, ethnicity. In our study, children in one-parent families were not more at risk of having enuresis, which is in contrast with previous work (Golding and Tissier 1986). It is possible that the cultural environment of one-parent families has changed; such families used to be very much a minority, but have become a common feature of society.

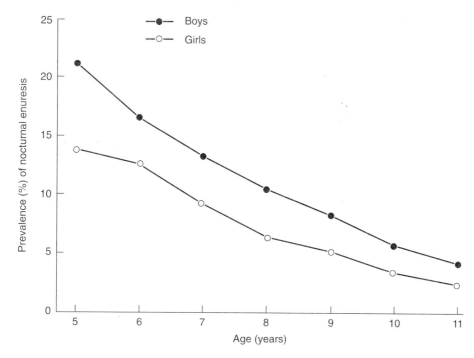

Fig. 12.2 Prevalence of nocturnal enuresis (more than once a week) by age and gender. Results taken from Rona *et al.* 1997*b*; with permission.

Disturbed sleep

In the NSHG we used a question developed by Clements and colleagues (1986). The parents were asked if their child had disturbed sleep at night, excluding periods of illness (Rona *et al.* 1998). The parents were presented with the following options: sleep disturbed most nights, cries, and needs attention; sleep disturbed once or twice a week, cries, and needs attention; sleep disturbed occasionally, cries, and needs attention; sleep disturbed, wants attention, but does not cry; sleeps poorly, but lies quietly when awake; and the child sleeps well. Disturbed sleep with a frequency of at least once a week decreased with age in both sexes reaching a prevalence of approximately 1% at the age of 9 years (Fig. 12.3). Poor sleep had a prevalence of 2% regardless of age or gender. The prevalence of disturbed sleep is in agreement with the results published by Pollock (1994) of 1.4% in 5-year-olds. However, studies in other countries tend to report higher prevalences of disturbed sleep (Kahn *et al.* 1989; Klackenberg 1982; Vela-Bueno *et al.* 1985). Although in part the discrepancy between studies may be due to the diversity of questions to assess disturbed sleep, the magnitude of the differences cannot entirely be due to questionnaire design. Along with Pollock (1994) we analysed sleep in a broader context while the other studies focused only on sleep problems. It would be important in future studies to reach an agreement on a standard questionnaire. Although of concern that 2% of children in the NSHG had severely disturbed sleep, and approximately 7% had occasionally disturbed sleep, the prevalences reported in the NHSG and the 1970 cohort (Pollock 1994) are not nearly as worrying as results published in other studies with percentages of over 30%. As the percentage of children with disturbed sleep decreased markedly with age it is probable that for a large percentage of 5-year-old children with disturbed

Table 12.3 Variables associated with enuresis after adjustment for confounders

Variable	n/N	OR (95% CI)
Ethnic group		
White (Scottish representative)	145/3742	1.00
White (English representative)	244/5788	1.04 (0.84–1.29)
White (English inner city)	113/1732	1.30 (1.00–1.69)
Afro-Caribbean	55/737	1.72 (1.22–2.42)
Indian subcontinent	72/2008	0.91 (0.66–1.94)
Birth order		
First born	200/4983	1.00
Second or third	323/6533	1.42 (1.17–1.72)
Fourth or later born	74/1647	1.43 (0.99–1.83)
Mother's age at child's birth		
<20 years	72/1096	1.00
20–24 years	232/4327	0.86 (0.65–1.15)
25–34 years	271/7095	0.61 (0.45–0.83)
≥ 35 years	45/1052	0.68 (0.45–1.04)
Sleep disturbed at night		
Sleeps well	505/12712	1.00
Sleeps poorly	12/223	1.32 (073–2.40)
Disturbed occasionally and cries	85/809	1.96 (1.53–2.51)
Disturbed ≥ 1 a week and cries	35/252	2.70 (1.85–3.96)
Mother's smoking at home (cigarettes per day)		
None	393/10146	1.00
1–9	54/1307	0.90 (0.67–1.22)
10–19	122/1082	1.58 (1.26–1.98)
≥20	61/857	1.60 (1.19–2.17)

Interaction of child's gender and father's social class not shown.
Taken from Rona *et al.* 1997*b*, with permission.

sleep the problem resolves itself over time. This was not seen among children with poor sleep, for which the percentage remained similar in all age groups.

Disturbed sleep, at least once a week, was more frequent in children of mothers with low educational level, in those exposed to maternal smoking, and in children of Indian subcontinent origin (Table 12.4). As for enuresis, several variables associated with social disadvantage are related to disturbed sleep. Curiously, the social variables related to disturbed sleep are different to those related to enuresis, except for maternal smoking.

There was also an association between enuresis and disturbed sleep. Children who had enuresis at least once a week had an odds ratio of 2.55 of having disturbed sleep in comparison to children without enuresis. Our study does not help to disentangle whether bedwetting causes disturbed sleep or the other way round. However, the level of association between the two problems is only moderate.

In our study we asked the parents to report disturbed sleep not caused by disease. In spite of this instruction a child with persistent wheeze was more likely to be reported to have severe disturbed sleep (OR 4.4). Disturbed sleep in children with clinical atopy was also reported by Pollock (1994)

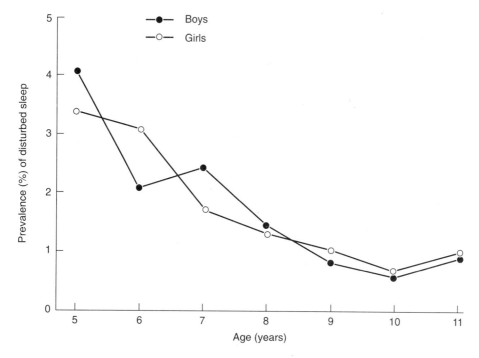

Fig. 12.3 Prevalence of disturbed sleep (at least once a week) by age and gender. Results taken from Rona *et al.*, *Archives of Disease in Childhood*, 1998, **78**, 20–5; with permission from the *BMJ* Publishing Group.

and in the ISAAC study (Pearce *et al.* 1993). It is possible that other chronic illnesses not explored in the NSHG may have also been the cause of sleeping problems in other children in the study.

Consultation with a doctor

Approximately 74% of the parents with a food intolerant child, slightly less than 50% of parents with a child with enuresis, and only 25% with a child with disturbed sleep or poor sleep consulted a doctor. The large differences in consultation with a doctor between the three conditions based on parents' perceptions is striking. The possible explanations for these differences may be related to the characteristics of parents with a child having one of the three types of disorder, to the parental perception of the severity of the disorder, to the perception that doctors can help, or to the level of the stigma attached to the condition.

Mothers of children with food intolerance were more likely to have had a higher education in contrast to children with disturbed sleep or enuresis. Enuresis and disturbed sleep were associated with social disadvantage and were more prevalent in ethnic minorities. The consultation rate was poorest for enuresis in the Afro-Caribbean group in which we found the prevalence to be the highest, while the consultation for disturbed sleep was lowest in those from the Indian subcontinent, despite the prevalence being the highest in that group. It is plausible then that family background is related to the probability of consulting for a medical problem. A contributory factor is that enuresis and disturbed sleep may not be perceived as severe problems by some groups, and in the case of enuresis it may also produce shame and embarrassment within the family.

Table 12.4   Variables associated with disturbed sleep at least once a week

Variable	n/N	OR (95% CI)
Nocturnal enuresis		
No enuresis	183/12026	1.00
< 1/month	18/930	1.03 (0.62–1.69)
⩾ 1/month and < 1/week	17/561	1.60 (0.95–2.68)
⩾ 1/week	38/672	2.55 (1.75–3.72)
Wheeze		
No wheeze	174/12129	1.00
Occasional wheeze	28/1412	1.43 (0.95–2.16)
Persistent wheeze	52/667	4.42 (3.17–6.13)
Ethnic background		
White (Scottish)	39/3783	1.00
White (English)	88/5788	1.25 (0.85–1.84)
White (English inner city)	34/1720	1.01 (0.62–1.64)
Afro-Caribbean	17/731	1.25 (0.68–2.30)
Indian subcontinent	63/1772	2.20 (1.34–3.60)
Mother's education		
College or university	44/3745	1.00
Secondary education	129/8140	1.14 (0.79–1.64)
Primary education or less	66/1467	2.41 (1.51–3.84)
Mother's smoking at home (cigarettes per day)		
None	162/9882	1.00
1–9	34/1316	1.93 (1.29–2.88)
10–19	30/1778	1.19 (0.78–1.83)
⩾ 20	23/855	1.87 (1.15–3.05)

Household overcrowding and father's social class were also significantly associated with poor sleep, due to the 'unknown information' category
Taken from Rona *et al.*, *Archives of Disease in Childhood*, 1998, **78**, 20–5; with permission from the *BMJ* Publishing Group.

Parents may perceive that health professionals are not good at tackling these problems. However, there is no good reason for thinking that doctors are better at tackling problems of food intolerance than enuresis or disturbed sleep. The effective elimination of food items to deal with food intolerance in the school-age group is laborious and not always successful. In relation to sleep disturbance it has been reported that advice given is often unhelpful (Kerr and Jowett 1994). Most children are prescribed sedatives, but Richman (1985) concluded that they were of limited use for dealing with the problem. Behavioural modifications have been recommended, but not all authors agree in their efficacy for treating disturbed sleep (Kerr and Jowett 1994). Alarm devices and desmopressin are considered efficacious for managing enuresis (Stenberg and Läckgren 1994; Thompson and Rey 1995), although the relapse rate is high (Forsythe and Butler 1989; Moffat *et al.* 1993). It is possible that the treatment of the condition is considered too laborious by many practitioners, but it is also possible that a large percentage of staff have limited knowledge of how to treat the conditions. In support of this explanation are the findings that 35% of the parents who consulted a doctor reported that the doctor did nothing and 40% remained unhappy with the management provided (Devlin 1992). The three conditions covered in this chapter are areas in which examples of good practice may help to address deficiencies and heterogeneity of service provision.

Conclusions

Severe illness in schoolchildren is relatively rare, but the frequency of health problems that cause distress in the family are not infrequent. We analysed three problems that are common in schoolchildren: food intolerance; enuresis; and sleep disturbance. The characteristics of the three disorders are different. Enuresis is the most common of the three, found in 5.5% of boys and 3.6% of girls, but the other two conditions are also frequent: 3–4% with serious sleep problems and approximately 2.8% with food intolerance. Food intolerance is reported more frequently in children of highly educated mothers, while enuresis and disturbed sleep are more frequent in children living in conditions of social disadvantage and in ethnic minorities. The demonstration that on average, food intolerant children are 0.3 SDS shorter than other children indicates that either these children genuinely have a health problem or current intervention by health staff or by the parents themselves may be damaging the child. The prevalence of enuresis has not changed over the last 45 years despite changes in the social environment. This indicates that behavioural manifestations of social disadvantage may be related to the aetiology of the disorder rather than material poverty itself. In relation to food intolerance and sleep disturbance there are few studies in the community, and it will be important to assess changes over time. There are reports in the literature that doctors are poor at dealing with the three health problems reported in this chapter. Examples of good practice may help to address the perceived deficiencies in the provision of services for these conditions.

13 Assessing the effect of changes in school-milk and school-meals policy over short periods of time

Background

The NSHG was prompted by changes in the governmental school-milk policy implemented in 1971. Although the committee responsible for its inception considered a randomized trial of milk provision this was deemed unfeasible (Department of Health and Social Security 1973). Furthermore, the NSHG began data collection in 1972, after the changes took place, so that even a quasi-experimental approach to evaluation was ruled out.

Readers interested in the history of the school-meals service before the Second World War are referred to an article by Ivatts (1992). The postwar changes in school-milk and school-meal provision are summarized in Table 13.1. Apart from the fact that changes in these two facets of welfare provision largely coincided there were many concurrent trends in social factors, notably unemployment rates, that might equally have been expected to affect child health and growth, and

Table 13.1 Provision of school milk and school meal prior to 1971 and changes during the period of the NSHG 1972–1994

	Time period	Statutory provision by Local Education Authorities
School milk:		
	1946–1968	All school pupils entitled to free one-third of a pint
	1968–1971	Primary and special-school pupils only
	1971–1980	Pupils under 7 years of age only
	1980–	No statutory obligation
	1983–	European Community subsidy available on milk
School meals:		
	Prior to 1971	Free school meals for children from families in receipt of Supplementary Benefit. Standard subsidized charge for others. Meal to be 'suitable as the midday meal' and provide one-third of daily nutrients and energy.
	1971—1980	Free school meals extended to families in receipt of Family Income Supplement. Subsidy decreased gradually.
	1980	Statutory requirement over content and universal provision of meal removed.
	1980–1988	Free school meals provided to children of families in receipt of Supplementary Benefit or Family Income Supplement.
	1988	Supplementary Benefit renamed Income Support, Family Income Supplement renamed Family Credit. Children of families receiving the latter lost their entitlement to free meals, but families received cash equivalent.

all of which are interrelated. Added to this are the difficulties in the analysis of height gain, as described earlier (Chapters 2 and 4). It is not surprising, therefore, that relatively few analyses were carried out to assess changes in milk and meals provision specifically. The analyses that were reported are described briefly under the two headings.

School-milk provision

Because the withdrawal of free school milk for children over 7 years of age was largely the reason for the NSHG being commissioned, the study team felt under an obligation to assess the effect as best they could. With height gain considered the most sensitive indicator of nutritional status the question was whether there were comparable groups of children with and without free school milk available. The Act laid down that free school milk should be withdrawn at the end of the term following the child's seventh birthday. However, from information supplied by the schools it was ascertained that the policy was not implemented in strict accordance with the Act (J. Cook *et al.* 1979). Not surprisingly many schools operated a class-based approach, supplying free milk according to the age of the majority of the children, but some schools followed the Act precisely, and a few continued to supply free school milk to all primary schoolchildren. Parental reports of the availability of free school milk corresponded with this information, and were used to define groups of children, over a 2-year period, for whom milk was available in both years, in neither year, or only at the first survey. For any pair of years only one cohort defined by year of birth contained substantial numbers in all three groups. For example, for 1972–1973 this was the cohort of children born in 1965, who became 7 years old either just before the 1972 survey or between the two surveys.

Height gain was compared between the three groups for the selected cohort, adjusted to a time gap of 1 year and 7 years of age at the first survey to allow for small deviations from the annual week of survey, and dependence of height gain on age. The alternative and preferable analysis of height at the second survey adjusted for height at the first, as well as for time gap and age, was also carried out. The analysis was performed for English and Scottish boys and girls, and four time periods, 1972–73, 1973–74, 1974–75, and 1975–76. Subanalyses were performed on data for children in manual social classes who might have been more likely to benefit from the availability of free school milk (J. Cook *et al.* 1979). No consistent relation was found, and parental reports indicated that almost all children drank milk at home. While the study could not rule out a benefit for the most deprived children in the population it was concluded that the effect of the availability of free school milk, if any, was very small.

No doubt government ministers used this as reassurance that the change in policy had had no deleterious effect. However, had lower rates of growth been found in the group without free milk available it would have been easy to explain this as due to confounding with area differences, an aspect which should have received attention in the paper.

Despite the initial view of the Sub-committee on Nutritional surveillance, that a randomized trial of milk provision was unfeasible (Department of Health and Social Security 1973), such a trial was carried out from 1976–1978 in 25 schools in Mid-Glamorgan, South Wales (Baker *et al.* 1980). Schools were selected for having at least 20% of children receiving free school meals, and within these schools 7- or 8-year-old children with at least three siblings were randomly allocated to receive one-third of a pint (187 mL) of milk daily for six school terms or to the control group. The average difference in height gain between the two groups over the period was 0.28 cm (95% confidence interval, 0.01–0.58 cm): 0.11 cm for boys and 0.45 cm for girls. The difference in weight gain was 130 g, and not statistically significant. The authors concluded that the effect was very small, and likely to be even smaller in the whole unselected population. In addition, it may be argued that an estimate from a randomized trial is likely to be greater than the effect of statutory provision.

Our first analysis essentially assessed the policy over the provision of milk, not the effect of the consumption of school milk. However, most children for whom school milk was available were reported to drink it. A second analysis was carried out for a 2-year period, from 1982 to 1984 for the English representative sample, from 1983 to 1985 for the English inner-city sample, and from 1982/83 to 1984/85 for the Scottish representative sample (Rona and Chinn 1989). There was considerable variation by then in the provision of milk at school: at the lowest, for around 25% of children, in the English representative sample and available predominantly to younger children; and highest, around 65%, in the inner-city sample. Almost all milk was free in the Scottish and inner-city samples, and was often available to older children, but in the English representative sample children in manual social classes were more likely to have the milk free, when available, than children from non-manual classes.

Children were divided in the second analysis on milk availability, rather than free milk availability, as there was no longer a uniform policy to be tested. No relation of milk availability to height gain was found.

School meals

There were two analyses also carried out to relate the rate of growth to whether the child took lunch at school. The first of these used data collected before the removal in 1980 of the statutory requirement over content and provision (Rona et al. 1983), and the second was carried out on data collected after 1980 in parallel with the second school-milk analysis outlined above (Rona and Chinn 1989).

Before 1980 there was a very marked difference in the uptake of school meals in England and Scotland. In England uptake was high, around 75%, and differed little between social classes. In Scotland it was lower and varied by social class, being around 55% for children of unskilled manual workers and 30–35% for children with fathers in non-manual and skilled or semi-skilled occupations. For the analyses of data from 1973 to 1979 (Rona et al. 1983) children were divided within each country into three groups according to a poverty index based on the fathers' occupation, number of siblings, and receipt of benefits by the family, and classified as 'poor', 'not poor', or 'undefined'. No consistent relation was found between the rate of growth and the uptake of school meals, even within the 'poor' group. Children in the 'poor' group were shorter than those in the 'not poor' group, with the undefined group being intermediate. Children who received a free school lunch were shorter than those who received a subsidized meal or had lunch at home, in other words the policy was targeted appropriately even if no effect on rate of growth could be detected. The relation between attained height and receipt of free school meals had been reported earlier (Rona et al. 1979), with the warning that proposed changes to the funding of school meals might prejudice the nutritional status of children receiving free school meals.

The analyses of the 1982–1985 data (Rona and Chinn 1989) also showed no relation of the rate of growth to lunch provision. Children in receipt of free school meals continued to be shorter than other children, in the inner-city sample as well as in the representative samples. Uptake of school meals had fallen in the English representative sample compared to the previous analysis, particularly in non-manual social classes, so that a social-class gradient in uptake was now evident.

Gulliford et al. (1991) did not report a relation of height to receipt of free school meals in the representative samples (Chapter 6), but social factors in the 1987 and 1988 data were analysed after adjustment for biological variables and family size, so this was not in conflict with the earlier findings that children in receipt of free school means were shorter.

Although in terms of the primary remit of the NSHG, namely to monitor the effect of changes in food policy on growth, nutritional, and health outcomes, it was not possible to detect direct effects,

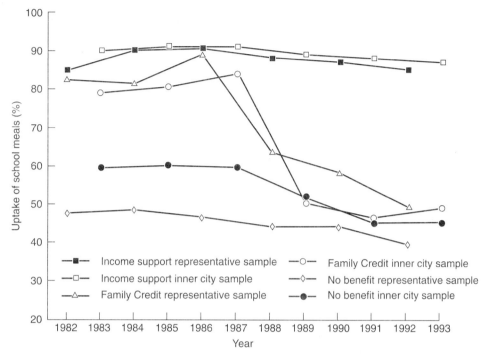

Fig. 13.1   The uptake of school meals by benefit group in the English representative sample and the inner-city sample. Before 1988, Family Credit was Family Income Supplement and Income Support was Supplementary Benefit. Taken from Somerville *et al.* 1996, with permission of the Oxford University Press.

the study was in a position to assess parental response to changes in policy. Questions on the uptake of school meals, social factors, and receipt of benefits were core items in the questionnaire (see Table 2.5), and in 1981 parental opinions were sought following the 1980 changes in provision. The price charged for a school meal was obtained from each school at the time of fieldwork, following the abolition of the statutory fixed price. The price of a school meal was the factor most strongly associated with uptake in England, with a trend towards decreased uptake over the price range of 40p, 45p, and 50p, and this was reflected in parents' expressed opinions (Rona and Chinn 1984*b*). In Scotland, the association was in the opposite direction, the higher price of 45p being associated with greater uptake than that at 40p. However, confounding of the price charged with other area characteristics that might influence uptake cannot be ruled out.

The NSHG could not offer a comprehensive picture of school-meal prices and uptake, but uniquely could provide information on uptake in relation to the receipt of benefits. In 1988, children of families in receipt of Family Credit, formerly Family Income Supplement, lost their entitlement to free school meals. Family Credit was increased by way of compensation (Somerville *et al.* 1996), but the uptake of school meals by these children dropped dramatically in both the English representative and inner-city samples (Fig. 13.1). In the latter sample, uptake before 1988 was lower by children of Indian subcontinent origin than by white or Afro-Caribbean children, irrespective of the benefits received, and the fall in uptake was greatest amongst Family Credit children in the Indian subcontinent group.

This demonstration of the large consequence of a financial change, even one designed to be neutral in its net effect, might have been expected to create considerable interest amongst policy advisers, nutritionists, and within educational authorities. As far as we know the findings had little impact, possibly because by their publication in 1996 they were seen as untimely.

Conclusions

The provision of free school milk was already in decline when the NSHG began data collection in 1972. School-meals provision was at its most favourable until 1980 (Ivatts 1992). As was seen in Chapter 4, the height of primary schoolchildren increased over the whole period, but we have no means of ascertaining whether the increase would have been greater if provision had not changed, or whether the growth of a small minority of particularly deprived children was impaired.

14 The public health perspective of the NSHG

The main public health problems in the nineteenth century were sanitation, housing, infection, nutrition, and the poor health and excess mortality of the population (Holland and Stewart 1998). By the beginning of the twentieth century these issues started to be tackled with some degree of success and, although these problems are still in evidence, the magnitude of their effects on health are comparatively minor in Britain today. To illustrate the magnitude of the changes that have occurred over the last century, infant mortality decreased from around 19% at the beginning of the century to approximately 6 per 1000 in 1996. The emphasis of public health activities changed and systems of health surveillance were adopted. Health surveillance was understood as the ongoing systematic collection of data, their constant evaluation, and dissemination to all who need to know to take remedial action, if needed (Langmuir 1976). In contrast to surveillance based on health events, the NSHG had its focus on biological characteristics of clinically normal subjects (Irwig 1976).

The NSHG surveillance system was centred on the accurate measurement of height, weight, and triceps skinfold thickness in a large number of children from a broad range of socioeconomic and cultural backgrounds. Overt undernutrition in terms of rickets was uncommon when the project was started, so that variation in the measurements between groups in society and changes over time became central in detecting deterioration or progress in the nutritional status of British children. It was also important to assess the impact of the government decision to change its policy over the provision of free school meals and welfare milk. There were several reasons behind this change. It was considered that standards of living, income, nutrition, etc. had greatly improved since the end of World War II. The problem, if there was one, was rather that of overnutrition. In addition, there was a great need to build new schools and improve the physical conditions for education, the school meals and welfare milk provision was expensive and it was considered by the politicians that better use could be made of these resources. In the 1970s this major change in welfare policy was opposed by many groups. Those concerned with health in general supported the change, as long as provision was made for those considered at highest risk and that a method be established that would enable adverse changes in growth, nutrition, and health to be identified while they were still mild, and that areas and populations put at risk by any such changes would also be identified (Department of Health and Social Security 1973), so that remedial action could be taken.

Reports were made at regular intervals (at least annually) to the Department of Health through the Subcommittee on Nutritional Surveillance, when meetings of this Subcommittee were frequent, and through its civil servants or publications in scientific journals thereafter. The initial observations reassured those responsible for the change in policy. Children continued to increase in stature, the withdrawal of welfare milk was not associated with any decline in growth, school-meal provision continued in all areas for those most in need, and the withdrawal of universal provision was not associated with a deterioration in nutritional status. The existence of the NSHG reassured some of those who had been opposed to the changes. The change in administration in 1974–75 led to no change in policy. I was told the policy was discussed in Cabinet and that our study was mentioned—and the study's findings reported to it—and that this convinced Cabinet to continue with the previous administration's policy.

The NSHG fully fulfilled the objectives set out by the Subcommittee on Nutritional Surveillance. It demonstrated that children in England and Scotland were increasing in height (Hughes *et al.* 1997); that the increase in height over time was greater in those ethnic groups who were shorter at the start of the study (Chinn *et al.* 1998*b*); and that the environmental component in the variation of height between children was small in comparison to biological components such as birthweight and parents' heights (Gulliford *et al.* 1991). We were unable to demonstrate that free school milk or subsidized school meals enhance growth (Rona and Chinn 1989). On the other hand the NSHG demonstrated a worrying increase in obesity in Britain (Hughes *et al.* 1997). Indeed, it demonstrated such an increase in terms of skinfold thickness well before any increment in the prevalence of obesity was shown in adults in Britain, and when little evidence of such an increase was available in the world literature (Chinn and Rona 1987*a*).

Although we continued to report our findings, interest had begun to wane. Our results aroused little concern either amongst the officials of the Departments of Health and Education, or the politicians. On only one occasion over the study period did the Chief Medical Officer's annual report include results from the NSHG (Department of Health 1988). The finding that amongst the majority of primary schoolchildren, particularly girls, obesity was increasing inexorably, with its possible long-term health consequences, was not considered worthy of attention—and even denied by a Secretary of State on one occasion. When a proposal to extend the surveillance programme to adolescent children, without an increase in cost, was submitted to the Department of Health, a reply was never received.

It is difficult for me to explain the reasons for this attitude, in spite of the fact that the originator of the system (Mrs Thatcher), was then Prime Minister. Possible explanations are that the findings were politically unwelcome at that time. A more likely explanation is, however, that there had been a change in those responsible for advising Ministers and responsible for public health policy. In the first 10 years of the NSHG most of those involved had had experience of the effects of nutritional deprivation before and during the Second World War. They thus had a keen interest in the findings of the NSHG and both understood and were concerned with the effects of poverty. Nutrition was also considered of great import in the maintenance and improvement of health. More recently, this concern has diminished because the effects of deficient nutrition on health have been less overt and those involved in public health have been more interested in the effects of overnutrition and its consequences on disease, such as coronary heart disease and diabetes, rather than generic effects on health and of poverty. Of course, the lack of concern could also be attributed to the deficiencies and lack of presentational and reporting skills by those responsible for the NSHG. Certainly no glossy brochures were ever produced. It is noteworthy that, although a number of papers from the NSHG were accepted for publication in the *British Medical Journal*, the main results of the programme met with less interest from the general journals and consequently were published in the specialist literature. This general lack of concern with nutrition and its effects on health is not limited to those to whom the NSHG team reported, but is common at all levels in medical education, and in clinical and public health organizations. Concerns with the effects of deprivation and inequality were also not prominent in the period 1980–1997.

The NSHG was originally designed to answer questions on nutrition. However, when the first field visits were made it was apparent that it could also be used to tackle other questions. Many of the areas included in the study at the start were in the North of England, where the measures of the Clean Air Act, 1956 to control air pollution were slow in being introduced (Department of the Environment 1976). Since there was concern to provide evidence that the Clean Air Act improved health, the opportunity was seized to assess this. The questionnaire included questions on respiratory symptoms. The majority of the children attending primary school lived within a 1-mile radius from the school. The schools and the local environmental health departments were easily persuaded to site air pollution monitors in, or very near, the school and thus a reasonable measure of exposure was obtained. A relationship between the levels of air pollution (smoke and SO_2) and the frequency of respiratory symptoms in the children aged 5–10 years was shown. With the introduction of the measures of the Clean Air Act over the next 5 years this association disappeared, thus demonstrating improvements in health (Melia *et al.* 1981*a,b*).

The ability to use the NSHG for examining other questions of child health has been exploited. I will illustrate this contribution with a few examples. The apparent increase in the frequency of asthma could be investigated because reliable, consistent measures of recording had been used in the same population over time. Thus it was shown that the increase in asthma in the UK was real, and not an artefact of changes in diagnostic practice (Burney *et al.* 1990).

Other questions, such as whether there is an effect of passive smoking on child health (Colley *et al.* 1974), were analysed on a much larger group of children than previously in the UK, and the results were convincing in demonstrating that passive smoking has an effect on respiratory morbidity in children (Somerville *et al.* 1988). It is rarely appreciated that the NSHG was a unique source of information on the health of ethnic minorities in Britain. Large samples of children were recruited from several ethnic groups. Thus it was able to provide authoritative information about the variation in nutritional status and respiratory illness between ethnic groups. For example, the NSHG illustrated underrecognition and undertreatment of asthma in children from ethnic minorities, but especially from the Indian subcontinent (Duran-Tauleria *et al.* 1996).

In the last years of the NSHG several risk factors for CHD in children, blood pressure level, serum cholesterol, and cardiorespiratory fitness, were studied. It is relevant from a public health perspective that fatness was consistently and highly associated with all these risk factors of CHD. The Bogalusa study in the USA also showed that of the factors measured in adolescents, obesity was the one factor most related to whether a parent had CHD (Bao *et al.* 1997). Thus it is possible to propose that the surveillance of obesity is an economic means for assessing the future possible risk of CHD in adults in place of other methods which are less acceptable to the community and more expensive, such as the continuous measurement of lipoproteins.

Conclusions

The NSHG provided an appropriate method of surveillance of nutritional status amid changes in welfare policy and socioeconomic circumstances. The method used involved close co-operation between schools, local health authorities, and the academic team. The measurements made were reliable and the quality control ensured comparability over time. The original intention had been for the academic unit to develop the methodology and that the study and system would be incorporated into the routine tasks of the OPCS (Office for Population Censuses and Surveys, now subsumed within the Office for National Statistics). However, the funds of the Department of Health were cut, and there was no opportunity for the system to be funded by the OPCS as a new venture. The Department, however, considered that the NSHG was a valuable resource in monitoring the health of schoolchildren. Continuation of funding for current activities was less difficult than a transfer to another agency and obtaining an increase in its budget. We were thus asked to continue the study.

For health surveillance it is essential that there is a reliable and repeatable set of relevant measurements available on similar populations over time. The system has to provide information in a timely fashion and action has to be taken on the basis of the results (Holland 1995). The NSHG satisfied all these criteria.

The problem with any long-term activity is to maintain the interest of the participants in the process, the workers involved in gathering data, and also those responsible for policy decisions on the result, and ensuring continuing funding. The participants in the process remained concerned. The interest of those collecting the data and its analysis was maintained by the ability to answer a wider range of problems than originally posed. Thus the NSHG was not only involved in monitoring nutritional status, but also contributed to a range of public health issues related to respiratory illness and lung growth, CHD risk factors, social issues with regard to welfare policy, and the epidemiology of conditions that make a great impact in family functioning such as nocturnal enuresis, disturbed sleep, and food intolerance.

The period of the study, 1972–1994, was also one of great political turmoil and disturbance amongst those responsible for public health (Holland and Stewart 1998). It is perhaps too much to expect that interest and concern is maintained for a surveillance system. Thus, when the NSHG began to indicate that welfare provisions for those in greatest need were becoming deficient (Somerville et al. 1996) this was an unwelcome message both to politicians and their policy advisers. The difficulties of maintaining funding, concern, and interest in long-term studies of public health significance is a major problem in our society. Whether a different attitude would have resulted if the NSHG had been part of an arm of a government agency is difficult to assess. However, with all these problems some conclusions can be drawn:

1. The system of surveillance adopted was able to provide both reliable and timely information, and was sufficiently flexible for new questions and concerns to be addressed.

2. Most difficult of all—but crucial—is that the public health community is sufficiently robust and concerned to insist on the maintenance of systems of health surveillance and is in a position to take action when necessary.

3. That the NSHG was able to collect reliable data on a large representative group of schoolchildren for 23 consecutive years is no small accomplishment. The findings of this study were a very important contribution to our knowledge and the development of health and clinical policies.

15 NSHG: the auxological perspective

Background

The science and practice of auxology divides fairly neatly into three parts. There is, first, science in the strict sense—characterization of the human growth curve, and its evolution and physiology. Second, there is the clinical-medical part—the use of measurements of the growth of particular individuals to monitor their health, to assess their recovery from disease or undernutrition, and to gauge the success or otherwise of a treatment. Third, there is the use of measurements of groups of children and youths, where samples from parts or the whole of a country's population are used to assess the economic and social well-being of those groups.

This third strand of the auxological rope has been called 'Growth as a mirror of the condition of society' (Tanner 1986) or, less grandly, auxological epidemiology (Tanner 1981). It is to this third strand that the National Study of Health and Growth has made such a strong and enduring contribution.

It was in the early part of the nineteenth century that this discipline of population growth studies appeared, born of the reaction of humanitarians to the appalling conditions of the poor and their children. It developed amongst the conglomerate of Factory Legislation, Poor Law Commissions, and Sanitation and Housing Acts, which embodied the new and powerful practice of Public Health. In Great Britain its progenitors were such remarkable men as John Fielding, Jeremy Bentham, Robert Owen, John Howard, and William Wilberforce; its pioneers were Nassau Senior, Edwin Chadwick, and William Farr. The results of the first measurements of children—all of the labouring class, some working in textile factories, others, the controls, working in other occupations—were presented to Parliament in 1833, in Chadwick's *Report of the Commissioners on the Employment of Children in Factories*. Some 4 years later a second, larger, survey was supervised by Leonard Horner, Chief Factory Inspector and first Warden (or Principal) of the University of London. The results of both are illustrated in Figs 15.1 and 15.2. The mean heights of these 9–18-year-old boys and girls were at or below the third percentile of the modern UK population, as were also their weights.

Things moved fast in the 1830s, and by the end of the year an Act of Parliament had been passed, controlling the worst malpractices of child labour. Strictly speaking, the impression that the growth of these factory children was stunted was an intuitive one, based presumably on the size of the legislators' own children. There were no measurements of not-working, middle-class children for comparison until the survey of Charles Roberts and Francis Galton in the 1870s. Figure 15.3 shows the social class difference at that time. Boys at Public (i.e. private) schools had heights around the present 25th percentile, while contemporary boys in manual workers' families were only slightly taller than those of 1833. From that day to this, epidemiological studies of growth have continued in an unbroken, though often tenuous chain, through the measurements in schools and infant welfare clinics, and the London County Council surveys of 1905–1965, to modern British growth standards and the NSHG.

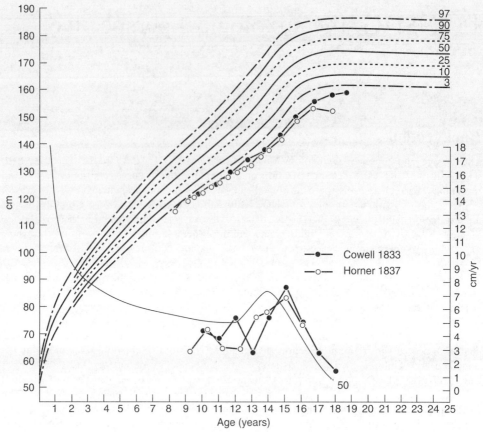

Fig. 15.1   Mean heights of boys working in factories in the Manchester–Leeds area in 1833 and 1837. Data plotted on British population standards of the 1960s. From Tanner 1981, with permission.

Achievement

In auxological circles, especially international ones, the NSHG has enjoyed an increasingly high reputation over the last 20 years. Perhaps this is chiefly because it has shown that with dedication, persistence, and a refusal to be discouraged by, at times, disdainful treatment from 'on high', the sort of continuous population-monitoring recommended by auxologists for many years can actually be done. The thing is possible: that is to say, at least schools covering the age range 5 to 11 years can be kept co-operative over long periods, pupils can be measured with a 95% compliance (certainly a world record), and the results can be processed and reported, on a continuous basis, within a year of the fieldwork (this is probably another world record). It is not the fault of the NSHG if the reports were for the most part pigeonholed; and it is a tribute to the international world of science and medicine that the results nevertheless found ready homes in the *Annals of Human Biology*, the *International Journal of Epidemiology*, the *European Journal of Clinical Nutrition*, and other journals.

Of course this is the easiest age group to monitor. The auxologist interested in the dynamics of growth and the interaction of growth rates with social conditions also needs studies of the

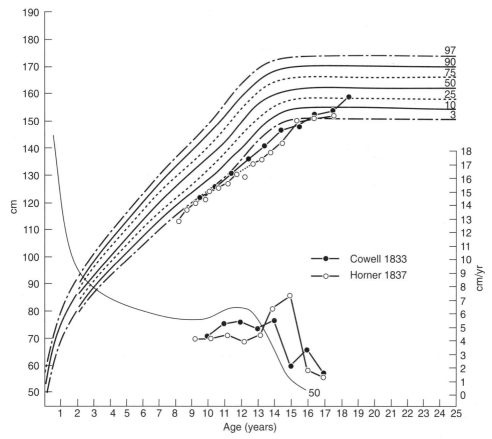

Fig. 15.2 Mean heights of girls working in factories in the Manchester–Leeds area in 1833 and 1837. Data plotted on British population standards of the 1960s. From Tanner 1981, with permission.

preschool age and of the pubertal and adolescent years. So much of the later course of growth is laid down in the early years, and so much greater is the plasticity then, that a monitoring system for the preschool period would be even more valuable. When the NSHG was set up this was fully realized, and a cognate study was arranged of children from birth to 5 years of age. Necessarily more restricted, this study nevertheless produced highly interesting results—the age by which differences in height associated with social class became significant for instance—but these were never placed in the public domain. As to the almost equally difficult period of 12–16 years of age, a proposal to integrate samples of adolescents into the NSHG was turned down, apparently for a lack of customer interest (Rona 1995).

Auxological issues

Surveys versus surveillance: populations versus individuals

Professor Holland has commented on the way public health issues were addressed by the NSHG. This was of course its main purpose, but there were strictly auxological issues arising and

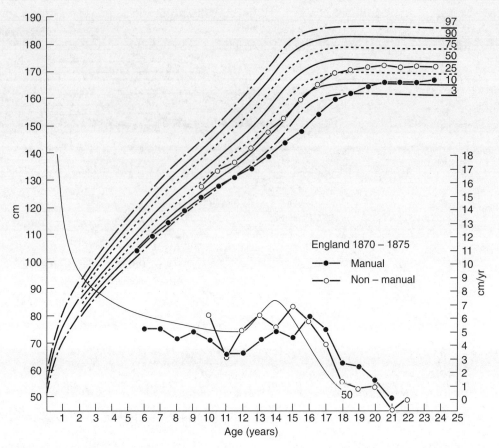

Fig. 15.3 Mean heights of boys by father's occupation (manual workers or non-manual, most professional, class) in about 1870 in England. Data plotted on British population standards of the 1960s. From Tanner 1981, with permission.

investigated too: the efficacy of a 10% overlap of measurements by school nurses and a highly trained anthropometrist in keeping the nurses' measurement reliability notably above what is expected in non-monitored schools; and the advisability of believing that the heights of husbands reported by wives are similar to the measured husbands' heights. But the chief auxological issues were those of statistical design and analysis.

Classical auxology studies of growth are divided into longitudinal, wherein the same child is measured repeatedly during all or part of her/his growth period, and cross-sectional studies, where all the individuals are measured once only, so that means at successive ages are each derived from different individuals.

Longitudinal studies are appropriate, indeed absolutely essential, for the study of the growth process, and all our knowledge of the intricacies and variations of the human growth curve is based upon them. Because of the variation in *tempo* of growth between children, some—the 'early maturers'—running through the whole growth process in a short span of years, others—the 'late maturers'—taking longer to reach, on average, the same result; because of this, and the fact that, especially at puberty, individuals have major departures from linearity of growth with time, at successive ages the means of cross-sectional data trace out a curve which is different from that of the typical or 'structural average' individual. This has been well known to auxologists for over a century, though it is still sometimes ignored today.

Cross-sectional studies, then, characterize no individual but the population or subpopulation from which they were drawn. Here we are not seeking to push forward the science of growth, our first auxological strand, but to exploit the social application of growth data, our third strand.

Many studies have combined longitudinal and cross-sectional elements: they have been called 'mixed-longitudinal'. In a basically birth-to-maturity longitudinal study, inevitably some children drop out, and others may be entered for the first time at various ages. It took many years before investigators making this type of study came to understand that analysing their data by just treating the longitudinal elements as though they were cross-sectional, and ignoring the individual's past and future, was a statistically inefficient thing to do (Tanner 1981). Special methods had to be used for estimating mean attained values for age, and especially mean increments from age to age (Tanner 1951).

The fundamental differences in use between longitudinal and cross-sectional studies have not always been well focused by investigators making growth studies. In the International Children's Centre Co-ordinated Longitudinal Growth Studies (see Tanner 1981) there was a tendency in some participating countries (France and Sweden are examples) to use their intensive, necessarily small-scale, studies not only to characterize differences between individuals but also to generate national growth standards, a clearly illegitimate use.

But should not some element of longitudinality be built in to a population surveillance study such as the NSHG, in which continuous monitoring was the point, contrasted with the many survey studies, in which simple cross-sections of the population were measured at intervals, usually of about 10 years?

One of the latest papers from the NSHG gives an important, perhaps paradoxical, answer to this question (Chinn 1995). The fundamental importance of distinguishing studies of individuals and studies of populations again emerges. When it comes to following individuals there is no dispute that the rate of growth (or increments) is a more sensitive indicator of current ill-health or undernutrition than height attained, which is only the initial screening tool. But Chinn points out that in population work it is far from clear that a comparison of the mean rates of growth of cohorts has an analogous advantage or indeed an analogous meaning. So it turns out that the longitudinal element in a surveillance programme is more of a complicating statistical nuisance than a public health advantage.

So next time do we revert to serial cross-sectional studies? Chinn thinks not, and for a social rather than a scientific reason. Due to the continuous nature of the project the response rate in the NSHG was of the order of 95%. In repeated random samplings of a population response rates are never this high: 80% is exceptional. This non-compliance irretrievably compromises comparability over time in successive cross-sectional surveys; whereas in the mixed longitudinal design the longitudinal element can be used to see if changes in compliance have had a differential effect.

Thus in the area of statistical design, the NSHG has made an important contribution to auxological epidemiology, all the more so by neatly balancing statistical method with human interaction.

The measurement of fatness

As in any branch of science, advances in auxology are often associated with the introduction of new tools, either physical or in the shape of statistical method. The NSHG was one of the first major population studies to use skinfold callipers to measure fatness, a technique long employed in intensive longitudinal studies.

When the Harpenden Growth Study began in 1948 the only callipers available were highly inaccurate and had a distressing tendency to fall to pieces, literally, in the operator's hand. They also had no way of compensating for the spring pressure being greater at large openings than at small ones. Then in about 1951 a young technician walked into the office of Tanner and Whitehouse with a form of dial-reading spring calliper used in his family business of leather merchandising. Modified to produce a constant pressure at all jaw openings, this became the Harpenden Skinfold Calliper, now in general use. The callipers required some skill to use however, and at first it was thought that only in the single-anthropometrist type of longitudinal study would they be acceptable. The NSHG changed that perception and introduced the skinfold calliper as the preferred method of assessing fat in childhood population surveys.

Second, the use of weight-for-height as a proxy for fatness has a history that goes back to Quetelet 150 years ago. But the distribution of height and weight make simple indices such as weight/height or weight/height^2 (kg/m^2)—the latter favoured by Quetelet himself—both inefficient and biased. In the NSHG a new index was computed giving values Normally distributed and homoscedastic over age, as well as independent of height: a desideratum of a generation of measurers. The index is $\log((\text{weight} - 9)/\text{height}^{3.7})$ and this predicted well the sum of triceps and subscapular skinfolds at the ages of 4–12 years. All the same, Hughes et al., in their summarizing paper on trends in growth (1997), warned that this index is less sensitive to an increase in fatness than the skinfolds, which in any future surveillance programme should be measured alongside height and weight.

Secular changes and the dynamics of the heredity–environment interaction

The NSHG followed subgroups of different ethnic origins to determine, of course, whether each was becoming more or less disadvantaged: this is 'growth as a mirror', precisely. But the dynamics of the changes amongst each of the groups over the 10 years 1983–1993 (Chinn et al. 1998a) may also throw light on one of the basic questions of auxology: to what extent are current ethnic differences in growth around the world simply the effect of environmental circumstances? This is a question that has been hotly, perhaps at times too hotly, debated over past years, admittedly mostly in relation to growth in the first 5 years of life (see Eveleth and Tanner 1990).

The NSHG followed representative samples of English and Scottish children, inner-city white children in deprived circumstances, as well as inner-city Afro-Caribbean, Punjabi, and Gujarati children. From the trends shown by each group we can derive some idea of the groups' approach to its genetically limiting height—at the ages 5–11 that is to say—under what we might call 'normal' Western European circumstances. Do the shortest ethnic groups catch up the representative? If not, are they at least approaching some end-point faster than the representative? And what end-point?

The representative English children increased the least: 0.85 cm per decade. Evidently in them the potential height under modern industrialized conditions is nearly reached. The Scottish representatives increased a little faster, so that one might suppose that their potential is likely to be the same as the English, to be reached, barring accidents, some 10 years on. Little room for genetic differences here, then.

The same is true of the Punjabis. But Gujarati children (though increasing faster, at about 2 cm per decade, in this rather small sample), are less tall than the other groups and at this rate would take 50 or more years to equal them—a strong argument for some remaining genetic difference. The Afro-Caribbeans increased at the same rate as the Scots; but they were not catching up the English representative sample, they were pulling away from them. So here we have a rather clear evidence of a genetic difference: Afro-Caribbeans are taller.

At least there are genetic differences at ages 5–11 years (see also Eveleth and Tanner 1990). It is a truism of auxology that height at this age reflects not only the final adult height, but the *tempo* of growth of the population: whether they are early maturers, like the Japanese, or late ones. Tall and advanced at 10 years of age may mean average or below at 18. *Tempo* differences between population subgroups have important social effects, perhaps more important than those attributed to height *per se*, but systematic data on that subject are left to the next programme of surveillance.

Appendix

The National Study of Health and Growth publications in chronological order

Altman, D. G. and Cook, J. (1973). A nutritional surveillance study. *Proceedings of the Royal Society of Medicine*, 66, 646–7.

Irwig, L. M. and Altman, D. G. (1974). Peak-flow meter and peak-flow gauge. *Lancet*, ii, 1325.

Altman, D. G. and Irwig, L. M. (1975). Men, women and obesity. *British Medical Journal*, i, 573–4. (Letter)

Irwig, L. M., Altman, D. G., Gibson, R. J. W., and Florey, C. du Ve. (1975). Air pollution: methods to study its relationship to respiratory disease in British schoolchildren. In *Commission of the European Communities, Health Protection Directorate, United States Environmental Protection Agency, WHO. Proceedings of the International Symposium on Recent Advances in the Assessment of the Health Effects of Environmental Pollution*, Vol. 1, pp. 289–300. 24–28 June 1974, Paris. Office for Official Publications of the European Communities, Luxembourg.

Irwig, L. M. (1976). Surveillance in developed countries with particular reference to child growth. *International Journal of Epidemiology*, 5, 57–61.

Melia, R. J. W., Florey, C. du V., Altman, D.G., and Swan, A.V. (1977). Association between gas cooking and respiratory disease in children. *British Medical Journal*, 2, 149–52.

Rona, R. and Altman, D. G. (1977). National Study of Health and Growth: standards of attained height, weight and triceps skinfold in English children 5 to 11 years old. *Annals of Human Biology*, 4, 501–23.

Holland, W. W., Beresford, S. A. A., Bewley, B. R., Florey, C. du V., and Rona, R. (1978). The very early recognition of coronary heart disease—epidemiology of risk factors in early life. In *Very early recognition of coronary disease* (ed. L. MacDonald, J. Goodwin, and L. Resuckov), pp. 3–10. Excerpta Medica, Amsterdam.

Leeder, S. R. and Holland, W. W. (1978). The influence of the environment on disease and growth in childhood. In *Recent advances in community medicine* (ed. A. E. Bennett), pp. 138–48. Churchill Livingstone, Edinburgh.

Rona, R. J., Swan, A. V., and Altman, D. G. (1978). Social factors and height of primary schoolchildren in England and Scotland. *Journal of Epidemiology and Community Health*, 32, 147–54.

Cook, J., Irwig, L. M., Chinn, S., Altman, D. G., and Florey, C. du V. (1979). The influence of availability of free school milk on the height of children in England and Scotland. *Journal of Epidemiology and Community Health*, 33, 171–6.

Melia, R. J. W., Florey, C. du V., and Chinn, S. (1979). The relation between respiratory illness in primary schoolchildren and the use of gas for cooking. I—Results from a National Survey. *International Journal of Epidemiology*, 8, 333–8.

Rona, R., Chinn, S., and Smith, A. M. (1979). Height of children receiving free school meals. *Lancet*, ii, 534. (Letter)

Rona, R., Wainwright, A., Altman, D., Irwig, L. M., and Florey, C. du V. (1979). Surveillance of growth as a measurement of health in the community. In *Measurement of levels of health* (ed. W. W. Holland, J. Ipsen, and J. Kostrzewski), pp. 397–404. WHO Regional Office for Europe, Copenhagen.

Chinn, S. and Morris, R. W. (1980). Standards of weight-for-height for English children 5.0 to 11.0 years. *Annals of Human Biology*, 7, 457–71.

Holland, W. W., Chinn, S., and Rona, R. J. (1980). The effect of cessation of free school milk. In *Symposium on nutrition, 1979, in the Royal College of Physicians of Edinburgh*. (ed. S. H. Davies), pp. 79–80. Royal College of Physicians, Edinburgh.

Holland, W. W., Chinn, S., and Wainwright, A. (1980). Weight and blood pressure in children. In *Childhood prevention of atherosclerosis and hypertension* (ed. R. M. Lauer and R. B. Shekelle), pp. 331–41. Raven, New York.

Rona, R. J. (1980). The National Study of Health and Growth (NSHG): surveillance on nutritional status of primary schoolchildren. *Health Visitor*, 53, 309–12.

Rona, R. and Florey, C. du V. (1980). National Study of Health and Growth: respiratory symptoms and height in primary schoolchildren. *International Journal of Epidemiology*, 9, 35–43.

Smith, A. M., Chinn, S., and Rona, R. (1980). Social factors and height gain of primary schoolchildren in England and Scotland. *Annals of Human Biology*, 7, 115–24.

Holland, W. W., Rona, R. J., Chinn, S., Altman, D. G., Irwig, L. M., Cook, J., *et al.* (1981). The National Study of Health and Growth. Surveillance of primary school children (1972–1976). In *Department of Health and Social Security Report on health and social subjects 21. Sub-Committee on Nutritional Surveillance: Second Report*, pp. 85–101. HMSO, London.

Melia, R. J. W., Florey, C. du V., and Swan, A. V. (1981). Respiratory illness in British schoolchildren and sulphur dioxide 1973–7. I: cross-sectional findings. *Journal of Epidemiology and Community Health*, 35, 161–7.

Melia, R. J. W., Florey, C. du V., and Chinn, S. (1981). Respiratory illness in British schoolchildren and atmospheric smoke and sulphur dioxide 1973–7. II: Longitudinal findings. *Journal of Epidemiology and Community Health*, 35, 168–73.

Melia, R. J. W., Florey, C. du V., Chinn, S., Goldstein, B. D., Brooks, A. G. F., John, H. H., *et al.* (1981). Indoor air pollution and its effects on health. *Journal of the Royal Society of Health*, i, 29–32.

Morris, R. W. and Chinn, S. (1981). Weight-for-height as a measure of obesity in English children 5 to 11 years old. *International Journal of Obesity*, 5, 359–66.

Rona, R. J. (1981). Genetic and environmental factors in the control of growth in childhood. *British Medical Bulletin*, 37, 265–72.

Rona, R. J., Florey, C. du V., Clarke, G. C., and Chinn, S. (1981). Parental smoking at home and height of children. *British Medical Journal*, 283, 1363.

Garman, A. R., Chinn, S., and Rona, R. J. (1982). The comparative growth of primary school children from one and two parent families. *Archives of Disease in Childhood*, 57, 453–8.

Melia, R. J. W., Florey, C. du Ve, Chinn, S., Goldstein, B. D., John, H. H., and Craighead, I. B. (1982). Children as a sentinel for respiratory disease in the United Kingdom. In *Environmental epidemiology* (ed. Paul E. Leaverton), pp. 59–66. Praeger, New York.

Rona, R. J. and Chinn, S. (1982). National Study of Health and Growth: social and family factors and obesity in primary schoolchildren. *Annals of Human Biology*, 9, 131–45.

Rona, R. J. and Chinn, S. (1982). Nutrition and social circumstances of primary schoolchildren. In *Nutrition and health a perspective: the current status of research on diet related disease* (ed. M. R. Turner), pp. 197–210. MTP Press, Lancaster.

Rona, R. J. and Morris, R. W. (1982). National Study of Health and Growth: social and family factors and overweight in English and Scottish parents. *Annals of Human Biology*, 9, 147–56.

Foster, J. M., Chinn, S., and Rona, R. J. (1983). The relation of the height of primary school children to population density. *International Journal of Epidemiology*, 12, 199–204.

Morgan, M. (1983). Measuring social inequality: occupational classifications and their alternatives. *Community Medicine*, 5, 116–24.

Morgan, M. and Chinn, S. (1983). ACORN group, social class, and child health. *Journal of Epidemiology and Community Health*, 37, 196–203.

Rona, R. J., Chinn, S., Marshall, B. S. M., and Eames, M. (1983). Growth status and the risk of contracting primary tuberculosis. *Archives of Disease in Childhood*, 58, 359–61.

Rona, R. J., Chinn, S., and Smith, A. M. (1983). School meals and the rate of growth of primary school children. *Journal of Epidemiology and Community Health*, 37, 8–15.

Chinn, S. and Rona, R. J. (1984). The secular trend in the height of primary school children in England and Scotland 1972 to 1980. *Annals of Human Biology*, 11, 1–16.

Rona, R. J. (1984). Ecological environment. Environment and physical growth: random comments on Ferro-Luzzi's overview. In *Proceedings of a NATO advanced study institute on genetic and environmental factors during the growth period, 1982, Brussels* (ed. C. Susanne), pp. 199–208. Plenum Press, London.

Rona, R. J. and Chinn, S. (1984). Parents' attitudes towards school meals for primary school children in 1981. *Human Nutrition: Applied Nutrition*, 38A, 187–98.

Rona, R. J. and Chinn, S. (1984). The National Study of Health and Growth: nutritional surveillance of primary school children 1972–81 with special reference to unemployment and social class. *Annals of Human Biology*, 11, 17–28.

Somerville, S. M., Rona, R. J., and Chinn, S. (1984). Obesity and respiratory symptoms in primary school. *Archives of Disease in Childhood*, 59, 940–4.

Rona, R. J., Chinn, S., and Florey, C. du V. (1985). Exposure to cigarette smoking and child's growth. *International Journal of Epidemiology*, 14, 402–9.

Rona, R. J. and Chinn, S. (1986). National Study of Health and Growth: social and biological factors associated with height of children from ethnic groups living in England. *Annals of Human Biology*, 13, 453–71.

Chinn S. and Rona, R. J. (1987). The efficiency of mixed longitudinal studies for measuring trends. *Journal of the Royal Society of Medicine*, 80, 544–6.

Rona, R. J. and Chinn, S. (1987). National Study of Health and Growth. Social and biological factors associated with weight-for-height and triceps skinfold of children from ethnic groups in England. *Annals of Human Biology*, 14, 231–48.

Chinn, S. and Rona, R. J. (1987). The secular trend in weight, weight-for-height and triceps skinfold thickness in primary school children in England and Scotland from 1972 to 1980. *Annals of Human Biology*, 14, 311–19.

Rona, R. J. and Chinn, S. (1987). Parents' perceptions of food intolerance in primary school children. *British Medical Journal*, 294, 863–6.

Rona, R. J., Chinn, S., Duggal, S., and Driver, A. P. (1987). Vegetarianism and growth in Urdu, Gujarati and Punjabi children in Britain. *Journal of Epidemiology and Community Health*, 41, 233–6.

Chinn, S. (1988). Mixed longitudinal studies: their efficiency for estimation of trends over time. *Annals of Human Biology*, 15, 443–54.

Melia, R. J. W., Chinn, S., and Rona, R. J. (1988). Respiratory illness and home environment of ethnic groups. *British Medical Journal*, 296, 1438–41.

Price, C. E., Rona, R. J., and Chinn, S. (1988). The height of primary school children and parents' perceptions of food intolerance. *British Medical Journal*, 296, 1696–9.

Rona, R. J., Chinn, S., and Holland, W. W. (1988). The National Study of Health and Growth (NSHG): nutritional status of children of ethnic minorities and inner city areas in England. In *Department of Health and Social Security Report on Health and Social Subjects 33. Sub-Committee on Nutritional Surveillance: Third Report.* HMSO, London.

Rona, R. J., Chinn, S., and Holland, W. W. (1988). The National Study of Health and Growth: surveillance and research into the growth of primary school children since 1972. In *Department of*

Health and Social Security Report on Health and Social Subjects 33. Sub-Committee on Nutritional Surveillance: Third Report. HMSO, London.

Somerville, S. M., Rona, R. J., and Chinn, S. (1988). Passive smoking and respiratory conditions in primary school children. *Journal of Epidemiology and Community Health*, 42, 105–10.

Chinn, S., Price, C. E., and Rona, R. J. (1989). The need for new reference curves for height. *Archives of Disease in Childhood*, 64, 1545–53.

Rona, R. J., Chinn, S., and Manning, R. (1989). The validity of reported parental height in inner city areas in England. *Annals of Human Biology*, 16, 41–4.

Chinn, S., Rona, R. J., and Price, C. E. (1989). The secular trend in height of primary school children in England and Scotland 1972 to 1979 and 1979 to 1986. *Annals of Human Biology*, 16, 387–95.

Rona, R. J. (1989). A surveillance system of growth in Britain. In *Auxology 88. Perspectives in the science of growth and development. 5th Congress of Auxology* (ed. J. M. Tanner), pp. 111–19. Smith-Gordon, London.

Rona, R. J. and Chinn, S. (1989). School meals, school milk and height of primary school children in England and Scotland in the eighties. *Journal of Epidemiology and Community Health*, 43, 66–71.

Burney, P. G. J., Chinn, S., and Rona, R. J. (1990). Has asthma prevalence increased in children? Evidence from the National Study of Health and Growth 1973–1986. *British Medical Journal*, 300, 1306–10.

Gulliford, M. C., Price, C. E., Rona, R. J., and Chinn, S. (1990). Sleep habits and height at ages five to eleven. *Archives of Disease in Childhood*, 65, 119–22.

Price, C. E., Rona, R. J., and Chinn, S. (1990). Associations of excessive irritability with common illnesses and food intolerance. *Journal of Paediatric and Perinatal Epidemiology*, 4, 156–60.

Chinn, S. and Rona, R. J. (1991). Quantifying health aspects of passive smoking in British children aged 5 to 11 years. *Journal of Epidemiology and Community Health*, 45, 188–94.

Gulliford, M. C., Chinn, S., and Rona, R. J. (1991). Social environment and height: England and Scotland 1987 and 1988. *Archives of Disease in Childhood*, 66, 235–40.

Rona, R. J. (1991). Nutritional surveillance in developed countries using anthropometry. In *Anthropometry assessment and nutritional status* (ed. J. H. Himes), pp. 301–18. Alan Liss, New York.

Rona, R. J. and Chinn, S. (1991). Father's unemployment and height of primary school children in Britain. *Annals of Human Biology*, 18, 441–8.

Chinn, S. (1992). A new method for calculation of height centiles for preadolescent children. *Annals of Human Biology*, 19, 221–32.

Chinn, S. and Rona, R. J. (1992). Height and age adjustment for cross-sectional studies of pulmonary function in children aged 6 to 11 years. *Thorax*, 47, 707–14.

Chinn, S., Rona, R. J., Gulliford, M. C., and Hammond, J. (1992). Weight for height in children aged 4 to 12 years. *European Journal of Clinical Nutrition*, 46, 489–500.

Gulliford, M. C., Rona, R. J., and Chinn, S. (1992). Trends in body mass index of young adults in England and Scotland from 1973 to 1988. *Journal of Epidemiology and Community Health*, 46, 187–90.

Hammond, J., Nelson, M., Chinn, S., and Rona, R. J. (1993). Validation of a food frequency questionnaire for assessing dietary intake in a study of coronary heart disease risk factors in children. *European Journal of Clinical Nutrition*, 47, 242–50.

Rona, R. J. and Chinn, S. (1993). Lung function, respiratory illness and passive smoking in British primary school children. *Thorax*, 48, 21–5.

Rona, R. J., Gulliford, M. C., and Chinn, S. (1993). Prematurity and intra-uterine growth: implications for respiratory health and lung function in childhood. *British Medical Journal*, 306, 817–20.

Somerville, S. M. and Rona, R. J. (1993). Respiratory conditions, including asthma, and height in primary school. *Annals of Human Biology*, 20, 369–80.

Chinn, S. and Rona, R. J. (1994). Trends in weight-for-height and triceps skinfold thickness in English and Scottish children 1972–82 and 1982–90. *Paediatric and Perinatal Epidemiology*, 8, 90–106.

Hammond, J., Chinn, S., Richardson, H., and Rona, R. J. (1994). Response to venepuncture for monitoring in primary school. *Archives of Disease in Childhood*, 70, 367–72.

Hammond, J., Chinn, S., Richardson, H., and Rona, R. J. (1994). Serum total cholesterol and ferritin, and blood haemoglobin concentrations in primary school children. *Archives of Disease in Childhood*, 70, 373–5.

Hammond, J., Rona, R. J., and Chinn, S. (1994). Estimation in community surveys of total body fat of children using bioelectrical impedance or skinfold thickness measurements. *European Journal of Clinical Nutrition*, 48, 164–71.

Rona, R. J. (1995). The National Study of Health and Growth (NSHG): 23 years on the road. *International Journal of Epidemiology*, 24, S69–74.

Chinn, S. (1995). Monitoring the growth of children: conclusions from a long-term study. *International Journal of Epidemiology*, 24, S75–8.

Duran-Tauleria, E., Rona, R. J., and Chinn, S. (1995). Factors associated with weight-for-height and skinfold thickness in British children. *Journal of Epidemiology and Community Health*, 49, 466–73.

Freeman, J. V., Cole, T. J., Chinn, S., Jones, P. R. M., White, E. M., and Preece, M. A. (1995). Cross-sectional stature and weight reference curves for the UK, 1990. *Archives of Disease in Childhood*, 73, 17–24.

Kikuchi, S., Rona, R. J., and Chinn, S. (1995). Physical fitness of 9 year olds in England: related factors. *Journal of Epidemiology and Community Health*, 49, 180–5.

Rona R. J. (1995). Monitoring nutritional status in England and Scotland. *In Essays on auxology presented to James Mourilyon Tanner*, pp. 291–302. Castlemead Publications, Welwyn Garden City.

Rona, R. J. and Chinn, S. (1995). Genetic and environmental influences on growth. *Journal of Medical Screening*, 2, 133–9.

Rona, R. J., Chinn, S., and Burney, P. (1995). Trends in the prevalence of asthma in Scottish and English primary school children 1982–92. *Thorax*, 50, 992–3.

Chinn, S., Cole, T. J., Preece, M. J., and Rona, R. J. (1996). Growth charts for ethnic populations in UK. *Lancet*, 347, 839–40. (Letter)

Duran-Tauleria, E., Rona, R. J., Chinn, S., and Burney, P. (1996). Does ethnicity influence asthma treatment in children? *British Medical Journal*, 313, 148–52.

Jones, C. O. H, Qureshi, S., Rona, R. J., and Chinn, S. (1996). Exercise-induced bronchoconstriction by ethnicity and presence of asthma in British nine year olds. *Thorax*, 51, 1134–6.

Rona, R. J., Qureshi, S., and Chinn, S. (1996). Factors related to total cholesterol and blood pressure in British nine year olds. *Journal of Epidemiology and Community Health*, 50, 512–18.

Somerville, S. M., Rona, R. J., Chinn, S., and Qureshi, S. (1996). Family credit and uptake of school meals in primary school. *Journal of Public Health Medicine*, 18, 98–106.

Bristow, A., Qureshi, S., Rona, R. J., and Chinn, S. (1997). The use of nutritional supplements by primary school children in England and Scotland: results from the National Study of Health and Growth. *European Journal of Clinical Nutrition*, 51, 366–9.

Hughes, J. M., Li, L., Chinn, S., and Rona, R. J. (1997). Trends in growth in England and Scotland, 1972 to 1994. *Archives of Disease in Childhood*, 76, 182–9.

Rona, R. J., Duran-Tauleria, E., and Chinn, S. (1997). Family size, atopic disorders in parents, asthma in children and ethnicity. *Journal of Allergy and Clinical Immunology*, 99, 454–60.

Rona, R. J., Li, L., and Chinn, S. (1997) Determinants of nocturnal enuresis in England and Scotland in the '90s. *Developmental Medicine and Child Neurology*, 39, 677–81.

Rona, R. J., Li, L, Gulliford, M. C., and Chinn S. (1998). Disturbed sleep: effects of socio-cultural factors and illness. *Archives of Disease in Childhood*, 78, 20–5.

Chinn, S., Rona, R., and Duran-Tauleria, E. (1998). Serum cholesterol and haematology at age 8 to 10 years. *Scandinavian Journal of Clinical and Laboratory Investigation*, 58, 135–42.

Chinn, S., Hughes, J. M., and Rona, R. J. (1998). Trends in growth and obesity in ethnic groups in Britain. *Archives of Disease in Childhood*, 78, 513–17.

Rona, R. J., Hughes, J. M., and Chinn, S. (1999). The association between asthma and family size between 1977 and 1994. *Journal of Epidemiology and Community Health*, **53**, 15–19.

Bettiol, H., Rona R. J., and Chinn, S. (1999). Variation in physical fitness between ethnic groups in nine year olds. *International Journal of Epidemiology*, **28**, 281–6.

Duran-Tauleria, E. and Rona, R. J. (1999). Geographical and socio-economic variation in asthma symptom prevalence in English and Scottish children. *Thorax* (In press)

References

Acheson, R. M. and Hewitt, D. (1954). The Oxford Child Health Survey: stature and skeletal maturity in the pre-school child. *British Journal of Preventive Social Medicine*, **8**, 59–65.

Adair, R. H. and Bauchner, H. (1993). Sleep problems in childhood. *Current Problems in Pediatrics*, **23**, 147–70.

Andersen, R. E., Crespo, C. J., Bartlett, S. J., Cheskin, L. J., and Pratt, M. (1998). Relationship of physical activity and television watching with body weight and level of fatness among children. *Journal of the American Medical Association*, **279**, 938–42.

Anderson, H. R. (1989*a*). Increase in hospital admissions for childhood asthma trends in referral, severity, and readmissions from 1970 to 1985 in a health region of the United Kingdom. *Thorax*, **44**, 614–19.

Anderson, H. R. (1989*b*). Is the prevalence of asthma changing? *Archives of Disease in Childhood*, **64**, 172–5.

Anderson, H. R., Butland, B. K., and Strachan, D. P. (1994). Trends in prevalence and severity of childhood asthma. *British Medical Journal*, **308**, 1600–4.

Armstrong, N., Balding, J., Gentle, P., and Kirby, B. (1990). Patterns of physical activity among 11 to 16 year old British children. *British Medical Journal*, **301**, 203–5.

Ashmore, M. (1995). Human exposure to human pollutants. *Clinical and Experimental Allergy*, **25** (Suppl. 3), 12–22.

Ayres, J. G. (1986). Acute asthma in Asian patients: hospital admissions and duration of stay in a district with a high immigrant population. *British Journal of Diseases of the Chest*, **80**, 242–8.

Baker, I. A., Elwood, P. C., Hughes, J., Jones, M., Moore, F., and Sweetnam, P. M. (1980). A randomised controlled trial of the effect of free school milk on the growth of children. *Journal of Epidemiology and Community Health*, **34**, 31–4.

Bakwin, H. (1971). Enuresis in twins. *American Journal of Disease in Childhood*, **121**, 222–5.

Balarajan, R. (1991). Ethnic differences in mortality from ischaemic heart disease and cerebrovascular disease in England and Scotland. *British Medical Journal*, **302**, 560–4.

Bao, W., Srinivasan, S. R., Valdez, R., Greenlund, K. J., Wattigney, W. A., and Berenson, G. S. (1997). Longitudinal changes in cardiovascular risk from childhood to young adulthood in offspring of parents with coronary artery disease. The Bogalusa heart study. *Journal of the American Medical Association*, **278**, 1749–54.

Barker, D. J. P. (1992) (ed.) *Fetal and infant origins of adult disease*. British Medical Journal, London.

Barker, D. J. P., Osmond, C., Golding, J., Kuh, D., and Wadsworth, M. E. J. (1989). Growth in utero, blood pressure in childhood and adult life, and mortality from cardiovascular disease. *British Medical Journal*, **298**, 259–62.

Barker, D. J. P., Winter, P. D., Osmond, C., Margetts, B. M., and Simmonds, S. J. (1992*a*). Weight in infancy and death from ischaemic heart disease. In *Fetal and infant origins of adult disease* (ed. D. J. P. Barker), pp. 141–9. *British Medical Journal*, London.

Barker, D. J. P., Godfrey, K. M., Fall, C., Osmond, C., Winter, P. D., and Shaheen, S. O. (1992*b*). Relation of birth weight and childhood respiratory infection to adult lung function and death from chronic obstructive airways disease. In *Fetal and infant origins of adult disease* (ed. D. J. P. Barker), pp. 150–61. *British Medical Journal*, London.

Berkey, C. S., Ware, J. H., Speizer, F. E., and Ferris, B. G. (1984). Passive smoking and height growth of preadolescent children. *International Journal of Epidemiology*, **13**, 454–8.

Bettiol, H., Rona, R. J., and Chinn, S. (1999). Variation in physical fitness between ethnic groups in nine year olds. *International Journal of Epidemiology*, **28**, 281–6.

Bland, J. M., Peacock, J. L., Anderson, H. R., Brooke, O. G., and De Curtis, M. (1990). The adjustment of birthweight for very early gestational ages: two related problems in statistical analysis. *Applied Statistics*, **39**, 229–39.

Blomfield, J. M. and Douglas, J. W. B. (1956). Bedwetting: prevalence among children 4–7 years. *Lancet*, **i**, 850–2.

Bodhurta, J. N., Mosteller, M., Hewitt, J.K., Nance, W.E., Moskovitz, W.B., Katz, S., *et al.* (1990). Genetic analysis of anthropometric measures in 11 year old twins: The Medical College of Virginia twin study. *Pediatric Research*, **28**, 1–4.

Bodzsár, É. B. and Susanne, C. (1998). *Secular growth changes in Europe*. Eötvös University Press, Budapest.

Boreham, C., Savage, J. M., Primrose, D., Cran, G., and Strain, J. (1993). Coronary risk factors in schoolchildren. *Archives of Disease in Childhood*, **68**, 182–6.

Bost, L., Primatesta, P., and McMunn, A. (1998). Anthropometric measures and eating habits. In *Health survey for England: The health of young people 1995–97* (ed. P. Prescott-Clarke and P. Primatesta). pp. 67–108. The Stationary Office, London.

Bransby, E. R., Burn, J. L., Magee, H. E., and MacKecknee, D. M. (1946). Effect of certain social conditions on the health of schoolchildren. *British Medical Journal*, **2**, 767.

Burney, P. G. J. (1997). Epidemiological trends. In *Asthma* (ed. P. J. Barnes, M. M. Grunstein, A. R. Leff, and A. J. Woolcock). pp. 35–47. Lippincott–Raven, Philadelphia.

Burney, P. G. J., Chinn, S., and Rona, R. J. (1990). Has the prevalence of asthma increased in children? Evidence from the national study of health and growth 1973–86. *British Medical Journal*, **300**, 1306–10.

Burns, T. L., Moll, P. P., and Lauer, R. M. (1989). The relation between ponderosity and coronary heart disease in children and their relatives. The Muscatine ponderosity family study. *American Journal of Epidemiology*, **129**, 973–87.

Burr, M. L., Butland, B. K., King, S., and Vaughan-Williams, E. (1989). Changes in asthma prevalence: two surveys 15 years apart. *Archives of Disease in Childhood*, **64**, 1452–6.

Campaigne, B. N., Morrison, J. A., Schuman, B. C., Falkner, F., Lakatos, E., Sprecher, D., *et al.* (1994). Indexes of obesity and comparison with previous national survey data in 9- and 10-year-old black and white girls: the national heart, lung, and blood institute growth and health study. *Journal of Pediatrics*, **124**, 675–80.

Carr, W., Zeitel, L., and Weiss K. (1992). Variations in asthma hospitalizations and death in New York City. *American Journal of Public Health*, **82**, 59–65.

Chandra, R. K. (1997). Food hypersensitivity and allergic disease: a selective review. *American Journal Clinical Nutrition*, **66**, 526S–9S.

Charlton, A. (1994). Children and passive smoking: a review. *Journal of Family Practice*, **38**, 267–77.

Chinn, S. (1988). Mixed longitudinal studies: their efficiency for the estimation of trends over time. *Annals of Human Biology*, **15**, 443–54.

Chinn, S. (1989a). Longitudinal studies: objectives and ethical considerations. In *Longitudinal studies. Methodology, growth and recent developments* (ed. E. A. Sand, C. Rumeau-Rouquette, S. Chinn, and J. Olsen). *Revue d'épidémiologie et de santé publique*, Special Issue, Vol. 37, pp. 417–29. Masson, Paris.

Chinn, S. (1989b). Changing exposure: passive smoking. In *Longitudinal studies. Methodology, growth and recent developments* (ed. E. A. Sand, C. Rumeau-Rouquette, S. Chinn, and J. Olsen). *Revue d'épidémiologie et de santé publique*, Special Issue, Vol. 37, pp. 499–505. Masson, Paris.

Chinn, S. (1992). A new method for calculation of height centiles for preadolescent children. *Annals of Human Biology*, **19**, 221–32.

Chinn, S. (1995). Monitoring the growth of children: conclusions from a long-term study. *International Journal of Epidemiology*, **24**, S75–8.

Chinn, S. and Morris, R. (1980). Standards of weight-for-height for English children aged 5.0 to 11.0 years old. *Annals of Human Biology*, **7**, 457–71.

Chinn, S. and Rona, R. J. (1984). The secular trend in the height of primary school children in England and Scotland 1972 to 1980. *Annals of Human Biology*, **11**, 1–16.

Chinn, S. and Rona R. J. (1987*a*). Secular trends in weight, weight-for-height and triceps skinfold thickness in primary school children in England and Scotland from 1972–1980. *Annals of Human Biology*, **14**, 311–19.

Chinn, S. and Rona, R. J. (1987*b*). The efficiency of mixed longitudinal studies for measuring trends. *Journal of the Royal Society of Medicine*, **80**, 544–6.

Chinn, S. and Rona, R. J. (1991). Quantifying health aspects of passive smoking in British children aged 5 to 11 years. *Journal of Epidemiology and Community Health*, **45**, 188–94.

Chinn, S. and Rona, R. J. (1992). Height and age adjustment for cross-sectional studies of pulmonary function in children aged 6 to 11 years. *Thorax*, **47**, 707–14.

Chinn, S. and Rona R. J. (1994). Trends in weight-for-height and triceps skinfold thickness in English and Scottish children 1972–82 and 1982–90. *Paediatric and Perinatal Epidemiology*, **8**, 90–106.

Chinn, S., Price, C. E., and Rona, R. J. (1989*a*). Need for new reference curves for height. *Archives of Disease in Childhood*, **64**, 1545–53.

Chinn, S., Rona, R. J., and Price, C. E. (1989*b*). The secular trend in height of primary school children in England and Scotland 1972 to 1979 and 1979 to 1986. *Annals of Human Biology*, **16**, 387–95.

Chinn, S., Rona, R. J., Gulliford, M. C., and Hammond, J. (1992). Weight for height in children aged 4 to 12 years. *European Journal of Clinical Nutrition*, **46**, 489–500.

Chinn, S., Hughes, J., and Rona, R. (1998*a*). Trends in growth and obesity in ethnic groups in Britain. *Archives of Disease in Childhood*, **78**, 513–17.

Chinn, S., Rona, R., and Duran-Tauleria, E. (1998*b*). Serum cholesterol and haematology at age eight to ten years. *Scandinavian Journal of Laboratory Investigation*, **58**, 135–42.

Clements, J., Wing, L., and Dunn, G. (1986). Sleep problems in handicapped children: a preliminary study. *Journal of Child Psychology and Psychiatry*, **27**, 399–407.

Cole, T. J. (1988). Fitting smoothed centile curves to reference data (with discussion). *Journal of the Royal Statistical Society A*, **151**, 385–418.

Cole, T. J., Freeman, J. V., and Preece, M. A. (1995). Body mass index reference curves for the UK, 1990. *Archives of Disease in Childhood*, **73**, 25–9.

Colhoun, H. and Prescott-Clarke, P. (1996). *Health Survey for England 1994. Volume I: Findings*, pp. 249–50. Joint Health Survey Unit. HMSO, London.

Colley, J. R. T., Holland, W. W., and Corkhill, R. T. (1974). Influence of passive smoking and parental phlegm on pneumonia and bronchitis in early childhood. Lancet, **ii**, 1031–4.

Committee for the Development of Sport. (1988). *Eurofit: European test of physical fitness*. pp. 30–9. Council for Europe, Rome.

Cook, D. G. and Strachan, D. P. (1997). Parental smoking and prevalence of respiratory symptoms and asthma in school age children. *Thorax*, **52**, 1081–94.

Cook, D. G., Strachan, D. P., and Carey, I. M. (1998). Parental smoking and spirometric indices in children. *Thorax*, **53**, 884–93.

Cook, J., Altman, D. G., Moore, D. M. C., Topp, S. G., Holland, W. W., and Elliott A. (1973). A survey of the nutritional status of schoolchildren. *British Journal of Preventive and Social Medicine*, **27**, 91–9.

Cook, J., Altman, D. G., Jacoby, A., Holland, W. W., and Elliott A. (1975*a*). The contribution made by school milk to the nutrition of primary schoolchildren. *British Journal of Nutrition*, **34**, 91–103.

Cook, J., Altman, D. G., Jacoby, A., Holland, W. W., and Elliott A. (1975*b*). School meals and the nutrition of schoolchildren. *British Journal of Preventive and Social Medicine*, **29**, 182–9.

Cook, J., Irwig, L. M., Chinn, S., Altman, D. G., and Florey, C. du V. (1979). The influence of availability of free school milk on the height of children in England and Scotland. *Journal of Epidemiology and Community Health*, **33**, 171–6.

Crane, J., Pearce, N., Shaw, R., Fitzharris, P., and Mayes, C. (1994). Asthma and having children. *British Medical Journal*, **309**, 272.

Cresanta, J. L., Srinivasan, S. R., Foster, T. A., Webber, L. S., and Berenson, G. S. (1982). Serum lipoprotein levels in children: epidemiologic and clinical implications. *Journal of Chronic Diseases*, **35**, 41–51.

Darke, S. J., Disselduff, M. M., and Try, G. P. (1980). A nutrition survey of children from one-parent families in Newcastle upon Tyne in 1970. *British Journal of Nutrition*, **44**, 237–41.

Davis, J. B. and Bulpitt, C. J. (1981). Atopy and wheeze in children according to parental atopy and family size. *Thorax*, **36**, 185–9.

Department of Health and Social Security (1973). *First report by the sub-committee on nutritional surveillance. Reports on health and social subjects,* No. 6, pp. iii, 10, 18–19. HMSO, London.

Department of Health and Social Security. (1981). *Sub-committee on nutritional surveillance: second report. Reports on health and social subjects* No. 21 p. 7. HMSO, London.

Department of Health. (1988). Health in the population: children. Children's growth and nutrition, pp. 74–81. *On the state of the public health for the year 1988.* HMSO, London.

Department of Health (1989). Report on Health and Social Subjects 36. *The diets of British schoolchildren,* p. 29. HMSO, London.

Department of the Environment. Central Unit on Environmental Pollution. (1976). Pollution paper No. 9. *Pollution control in Great Britain: How it works*, pp. 9–10. HMSO, London.

De Swiet, M., Fayers, P., and Shinebourne, E. A. (1992). Blood pressure in the first 10 years of life. *British Medical Journal*, **304**, 23–6.

Devlin, J. B. (1992). Prevalence and risk factors for childhood nocturnal enuresis. *Irish Medical Journal*, **18**, 118–20.

Dockery, D. W., Berkey, C. S., Ware, J. H., Speizer, F. E., and Ferris, B. G. (1983). Distribution of forced vital capacity and forced expiratory volume in one second in children 6 to 11 years of age. *American Review of Respiratory Disease*, **128**, 405–12.

Dong, W., Primatesta, P., and Bost, L. (1998). Blood pressure. In *Health survey for England 1996. Volume I: Findings* (ed. P. Prescott-Clarke and P. Primatesta), Chapter 6, pp. 241–79. HMSO, London.

Duran-Tauleria, E. and Rona, R. J. (1999). Geographical and socio-economic variation in asthma symptom prevalence in English and Scottish children. *Thorax* (In press.)

Duran-Tauleria, E., Rona, R. J., and Chinn, S. (1995). Factors associated with weight for height and skinfold thickness in British children. *Journal of Epidemiology and Community Health*, **49**, 466–73.

Duran-Tauleria, E., Rona, R. J., Chinn, S., and Burney, P. (1996). Influence of ethnic group on asthma treatment in children in 1990–1: national cross sectional study. *British Medical Journal*, **313**, 148–52.

Emberlin, J., Savage, M., and Jones, S. (1993). Annual variations in grass pollen seasons in London 1961–1990; trends and forecast models. *Clinical and Experimental Allergy*, **23**, 911–18.

Essen, J. and Peckham, C. (1976). Nocturnal enuresis in childhood. *Developmental Medicine and Child Neurology*, **18**, 577–89.

Eveleth, P. B. and Tanner, J. M. (1976). *Worldwide variation in human growth* (1st edn), pp. 16–18, 52–3. Cambridge University Press, Cambridge.

Eveleth, P. B. and Tanner, J. M. (1990). *Worldwide variation in human growth* (2nd edn), pp. 89, 176–90, Cambridge University Press, Cambridge.

Fergusson, D. M., Horwood, L. J., Shannon, F. T., and Taylor, B. (1981). Parental smoking and lower respiratory illness in the first three years of life. *Journal of Epidemiology and Community Health*, **35**, 180–4.

Forsythe, W. I. and Butler R. J. (1989). Fifty years of enuretic alarms. *Archives of Disease in Childhood*, **64**, 879–85.

Foster, J. M., Chinn, S., and Rona, R. J. (1983). The relation of the height of primary school children to population density. *International Journal of Epidemiology*, **66**, 235–40.

Foster, T. A., Webber, L. S., Srinivasan, S. R., Voors, A. W., and Berenson, G. (1980). Measurement error of risk factor variables in an epidemiologic study of children—the Bogalusa heart study. *Journal of Chronic Disease*, **33**, 661–72.

Freedman, D. S., Srinivasan, S. R., Cresanta, J. L., Webber, L. S., and Berenson G. S. (1987). Serum lipids and lipoproteins. *Pediatrics*, **80** (supplement), 78–96.

Freedman, D. S., Srinivasan, S. R., Valdez, R. A., Williamson, D. F., and Berenson, G. S. (1997). Secular increases in relative weight and adiposity among children over two decades: the Bogalusa heart study. *Pediatrics*, **99**, 420–6.

Freeman, J. V., Cole, T. J., Chinn, S., Jones, P. R. M., White, E. M., and Preece, M. A. (1995). Cross-sectional stature and weight reference curves for the UK, 1990. *Archives of Disease in Childhood*, **73**, 17–24.

Garman, A. R., Chinn, S., and Rona, R. J. (1982). The comparative growth of primary school children from one and two parent families. *Archives of Disease in Childhood*, **57**, 453–8.

Gassner, M. (1992). Immunologische-allergologische Reaktionen unter veranderten Umweltbedungingen. *Schweizerische Rundschau fur Medizin/Praxis*, **81**, 426–30.

Gergen, P. J. and Weiss, K. B. (1990). Changing patterns of asthma hospitalization among children: 1979 to 1987. *Journal of the American Medical Association*, **264**, 1688–92.

Gidding, S. S., Bao, W., Srinivasan, S. R., and Berenson, G. S. (1995). Effects of secular trends in obesity on coronary risk factors in children: The Bogalusa Heart Study. *Journal of Pediatrics*, **127**, 868–74.

Golding, J. and Tissier, G. (1986). Soiling and wetting. In *From birth to five. A study of the health and behaviour of Britain's 5 year-olds* (ed. N. R. Butler and J. Golding), pp. 64–79. Pergamon, Oxford.

Goldstein, H. (1971). Factors influencing the height of seven-old-children: results from the National Child Development Study. *Human Biology*, **43**, 92–111.

Goldstein, H. and Tanner, J. M. (1980). Ecological considerations in the creation and use of child growth standards. *The Lancet*, **i**, 582–5.

Gortmaker, S. L., Dietz, W. H., Sobol, A. M., and Wehler, C. A. (1987). Increasing pediatric obesity in the United States. *American Journal of Disease in Childhood*, **141**, 535–40.

Groll, A., Preece, M. A., Candy, D. C. A., and Tanner, J. M. (1980). Short stature as the primary manifestation of coeliac disease. *Lancet*, **i**, 1097–9.

Gulliford, M. C., Price, C. E., Rona, R. J., and Chinn, S. (1990). Sleep habits and height at 5 to 11. *Archives of Disease in Childhood*, **65**, 119–22.

Gulliford, M. C., Chinn, S., and Rona, R. J. (1991). Social environment and height: England and Scotland 1987 and 1988. *Archives of Disease in Childhood*, **66**, 235–40.

Guyatt, G. H. and Newhouse, M. T. (1985). Are active and passive smoking harmful? determining causation. *Chest*, **88**, 445–51.

Hammond, J., Chinn, S., Richardson, H., and Rona, R. (1994*a*). Response to venepuncture for monitoring in primary school. *Archives of Disease in Childhood*, **70**, 367–72.

Hammond, J., Rona, R. J., and Chinn, S. (1994*b*). Estimation in community surveys of total body fat of children using bioelectrical impedance or skinfold thickness measurements. *European Journal of Clinical Nutrition*, **48**, 164–71.

Hammond, J., Chinn, S., and Rona, R. J. (1994*c*). Serum total cholesterol and ferritin and blood haemoglobin concentrations in primary schoolchildren. *Archives of Disease in Childhood*, **70**, 373–5.

Harlan, W. R., Landis, J. R., Flegal, K. M., Davis, C. S., and Miller, M. E. (1988). Secular trends in body mass in the United States 1960–1980. *American Journal of Epidemiology*, **128**, 1065–74.

Hasselblad, V., Humble, C. G., Graham, M. G., and Anderson, H. S. (1981). Indoor environmental determinants of lung function. *American Review of Respiratory Disease*, **123**, 479–85.

Hauspie, R., Susanne, C., and Alexander, F. (1977). Maturational delay and temporal growth retardation in asthmatic boys. *Journal of Allergy and Clinical Immunology*, **59**, 200–6.

Hay, I. F. C. and Higginbottam, T. C. (1987). Has the management of asthma improved? *Lancet*, **ii**, 609–11.

Hill, R. A., Standen, P. J., and Tattersfield, A. E. (1989a). Asthma, wheezing, and school absence in primary schools. *Archives of Disease in Childhood*, **64**, 246–51.

Hill, R., Williams, J., Tattersfield, A., and Britton, J. R. (1989b). Change in use of asthma as a diagnostic label for wheezing illness in schoolchildren. *British Medical Journal*, **299**, 898.

Holland, W. W. (1995). Achieving an ethical health service: the need for information. *Journal of the Royal College of Physicians of London*, **29**, 325–334.

Holland, W. W. and Beresford, S. A. A. (1974). Factors influencing blood pressure in children. In *Epidemiology and control of hypertension* (ed. O. Paul), pp. 375–86. Symposia Specialist, London.

Holland, W. W. and Stewart, S. (1998). *Public health. The vision and the challenge*. The Rock Carling Fellowship 1997. The Nuffield Trust, London.

Holland, W. W., Halil, T., Bennett A. E., and Elliott A. (1969). Factors influencing the onset of chronic respiratory disease. *British Medical Journal*, **2**, 205–8.

Howe, P. E. and Schiller, M. (1952). Growth responses of the schoolchild to changes in diet and environmental factors. *Journal of Applied Physiology*, **5**, 51.

Hughes, J. M., Chinn, S., and Rona, R. J. (1997). Trends in growth in England and Scotland 1972 to 1994. *Archives of Disease in Childhood*, **76**, 182–9.

Hunter, W. M. and Rigal, W. M. (1966). The diurnal pattern of plasma growth hormone concentration in children and adolescents. *Journal of Endocrinology*, **34**, 147–53.

Irwig, L. M. (1976). Surveillance in developed countries with particular reference to child growth. *International Journal of Epidemiology*, **5**, 57–61.

Ivatts, J. (1992). The case of the school meals service. *Social Policy and Administration*, **26**, 227–44.

Jacoby, A., Altman, D. G., Cook, J., Holland, W. W., and Elliott, A. (1975). Influence of some social and environmental factors on the nutrient intake and nutritional status of schoolchildren. *British Journal of Preventive and Social Medicine*, **29**, 116–20.

Jarvis, D., Luczynska, C., Chinn, S., and Burney, P. (1995). The association of age, gender and smoking with total IgE and specific IgE. *Clinical and Experimental Allergy*, **25**, 1083–91.

Jarvis, D., Chinn, S., Luczynska, C., and Burney, P. (1996). Association of respiratory symptoms and lung function in young adults with use of domestic appliances. *Lancet*, **347**, 426–31.

Jarvis, D., Chinn, S., Luczynska, C., and Burney, P. (1997). The association of family size with atopy and atopic disease. *Clinical and Experimental Allergy*, **27**, 240–5.

Johnston, I. D. A., Bland, J. M., and Anderson, H. R. (1987). Ethnic variation in respiratory morbidity and lung function variation in childhood. *Thorax*, **42**, 542–8.

Jones, O. H., Qureshi, S., Rona, R. J., and Chinn, S. (1996). Exercise-induced bronchoconstriction by ethnicity and presence of asthma in British nine year olds. *Thorax*, **51**, 1134–6.

Kahn, A., Merckt, C. Van de, Rebuffat, E., Mozin, M. J., Soltiaux, M., Blum, D., *et al.* (1989). Sleep problems in healthy pre-adolescents. *Pediatrics*, **84**, 542–6.

Kaplan, T. A. and Montana, E. (1993). Exercise-induced bronchospasm in nonasthmatic obese children. *Clinical Pediatrics*, **32**, 220–5.

Kerr, S. and Jowett, S. (1994). Sleep problems in pre-school children: a review of the literature. *Child: Care, Health and Development*, **20**, 379–91.

Kesteloot, H. and Joossens, J. V. (1992). Nutrition and international patterns of disease. In *Coronary heart disease epidemiology* (ed. M. Marmot and P. Elliott), Chapter 11, pp. 152–65. Oxford University Press, Oxford.

Kikuchi, S., Rona, R. J., and Chinn, S. (1995). Physical fitness of 9 year olds in England: related factors. *Journal of Epidemiology and Community Health*, **49**, 180–5.

Klackenberg, G. (1982). Sleep behaviour studied longitudinally: data from 14–16 years on duration, night-awakening and bed sharing. *Acta Paediatrica Scandinavica*, **71**, 501–6.

Knuiman, J. T., Hermus, R. J. J., and Hautvast, J. A. J. G. (1980). Serum total and high density lipoprotein (HDL) cholesterol concentrations in rural and urban boys from 16 countries. *Atherosclerosis*, **36**, 529–37.

Kuskowska-Wolk, A. and Bergstrom, R. (1993). Trends in body mass index and prevalence of obesity in Swedish men 1980–89. *Journal of Epidemiology and Community Health*, **47**, 103–8.

Lake, J. K., Power, C., and Cole, T. J. (1997). Child to adult body mass index in the 1958 British birth cohort: associations with parental obesity. *Archives of Disease in Childhood*, **77**, 376–81.

Langmuir, A. D. (1976). William Farr: Founder of modern concepts of surveillance. *International Journal of Epidemiology*, **5**, 13–18.

Lapidus, L., Bergtsson, C., Larsson, B., Pennert, K., Rybo, E., and Sjostrom, L. (1984). Distribution of adipose tissue and risk of cardiovascular disease and death: a 12 year follow up of participants in the population study of women in Gothenburg, Sweden. *British Medical Journal*, **289**, 1257–61.

Lauer, R. M., Burns, T. L., Clarke, W. R., and Magoney, L. T. (1991). Childhood prediction of future blood pressure. *Hypertension*, **18** (supplement I), 74–81.

Law, C. M., De Swiet, M., Osmond, C., Fayers, P. M., Barker, D. J. P., Cruddas, A. M., *et al.* (1993). Initiation of hypertension in utero and its amplification throughout life. *British Medical Journal*, **306**, 24–7.

Lebowitz, M. D. and Holberg, C. J. (1988). Effects of parental smoking and other risk factors on the development of pulmonary function in children and adolescents. *American Journal of Epidemiology*, **128**, 589–97.

Lebowitz, M. D., Holberg, C. J., Knudson, R. J., and Burrows, B. (1987). Longitudinal study of lung function development in childhood, adolescence and early adulthood. *American Review of Respiratory Disease*, **136**, 69–75.

Leeder, S. R., Corkhill, R., Irwig, L. M., Holland, W. W., and Colley, J. R. T. (1976). Influence of family factors on the incidence of lower respiratory illness during the first year of life. *British Journal of Preventive and Social Medicine*, **30**, 203–12.

Lewis, S., Butland, B., Strachan, D., Bynner, J., Richards, D., Butler, N., *et al.* (1996). Study of the aetiology of wheezing illness at age 16 in two national British birth cohorts. *Thorax*, **51**, 670–6.

Luczynska, C. M., Li, Y., Chapman, M. D., and Platts-Mills, T. (1990). Airborne concentrations and particle size distribution of allergen derived from domestic cats (*Felis domesticus*); measurements using a cascade impactor, liquid impinger and a two site monoclonal antibody for Fel d1. *American Review of Respiratory Disease*, **141**, 361–7.

Luder E., Melnik, T. A., and DiMaio, M. (1998). Association of being overweight with greater asthma symptoms in inner city black Hispanic children. *Journal of Pediatrics*, **132**, 699–703.

Magnusson, C. G. (1986). Maternal smoking influences cord serum IgE and IgD levels and increases the risk for subsequent infant allergy. *Journal of Allergy and Clinical Immunology*, **78**, 898–904.

Mann G. V., Pearson, G., Gordon, T., and Dawber, T. R. (1962). Diet and cardiovascular disease in the Framingham study. I Measurement of dietary intake. *American Journal of Clinical Nutrition*, **11**, 200–25.

Marr, J. W. (1971). Individual dietary surveys: purposes and methods. *World Review of Nutrition and Dietetics*, **13**, 105–64.

Melia, R. J. W., Florey, C. du V., Altman, D. G., and Swan, A. V. (1977). Association between gas cooking and respiratory disease in children. *British Medical Journal*, **2**, 149–52.

Melia, R. J., Florey, C. du V., and Chinn, S. (1979). The relation between respiratory illness in primary schoolchildren and the use of gas for cooking. I—Results from a national survey. *International Journal of Epidemiology*, **8**, 333–8.

Melia, R. J. W., Florey, C. du V., and Swan, A. V. (1981*a*). Respiratory illness in British schoolchildren and atmospheric smoke and sulphur dioxide 1973–7. I: Cross-sectional findings. *Journal of Epidemiology and Community Health*, **35**, 161–7.

Melia, R. J. W., Florey, C. du V., and Chinn, S. (1981*b*). Respiratory illness in British schoolchildren and atmospheric smoke and sulphur dioxide 1973–7. II: Longitudinal findings. *Journal of Epidemiology and Community Health*, **35**, 168–73.

Melia, R. J. W., Chinn, S., and Rona, R. J. (1988). Respiratory illness and home environment of ethnic groups. *British Medical Journal*, **296**, 1438–41.

Mielck, A., Retmeir, P., and Wjst, M. (1996). Severity of childhood asthma by socioeconomic status. *International Journal of Epidemiology*, **25**, 388–93.

Miller, F. J. W., Court, S. D. M., Knox, E. G., and Brandon, S. (1974). *The school years in Newcastle-upon-Tyne*, pp. 152–61. Oxford University Press, Oxford.

Moffat, M. E. K., Harlos, S., Kirshen, A. J., and Burd, L. (1993). Desmopressin acetate and nocturnal enuresis: how much do we know? *Pediatrics*, **92**, 420–5.

Morris, R. W. and Chinn, S. (1981). Weight-for-height as a measure of obesity in English children five to 11 years old. *International Journal of Obesity*, **5**, 359–66.

Morrison Smith, J. (1976). The prevalence of asthma and wheezing in children. *British Journal of Diseases of the Chest*, **70**, 73–7.

Moser, C. A. and Kalton, G. (1971). *Survey methods in social investigation*, pp. 100–11. Heinemann, London.

Nakagomi, T., Itaya, H., Tominaga, T., Yamaki, M., Hisamatsu, S-I., and Nakagomi, O. (1994). Is atopy increasing? *Lancet*, **343**, 121–2 (letter).

Negri, E., Pagano, R., Decarli, A., and La Vecchia, C. (1988). Body weight and the prevalence of chronic diseases. *Journal of Epidemiology and Community Health*, **42**, 24–9.

Nelson, M. and Bingham, S. A. (1997). Assessment of food consumption and nutrient intake. Past intake. In *Design concepts in nutritional epidemiology* (2nd edn) (ed. B. M. Margetts and M. Nelson), pp. 123–69. Oxford University Press, Oxford.

Ninan, T. K. and Russell, G. (1992). Respiratory symptoms and atopy in Aberdeen schoolchildren: evidence from two surveys 25 years apart. *British Medical Journal*, **304**, 873–5.

Omenaas, E., Bakke, P., Elsayed, S., Hanoa, R., and Gulsvik, A. (1994). Total and specific serum IgE levels in adults: relationship to sex, age and environmental factors. *Clinical and Experimental Allergy*, **24**, 530–9.

Office for Population Census and Surveys (OPCS) (1987). *Birth statistics*. OPCS Series FM1 no. 13. HMSO, London.

Pararajasingam, C. D., Sittampalam, L., Damani, P., Pattermore, P. K., and Holgate, S.T. (1992). Comparison of the prevalence of asthma among Asian and European children in Southampton. *Thorax*, **47**, 529–32.

Patrick, J. M. and Patel, A. (1986). Ethnic differences in the growth of lung function in children: a cross sectional study in inner city Nottingham. *Annals of Human Biology*, **13**, 307–15.

Pearce, N., Weiland, S., Keil, U., Langridge, P., Anderson, H. R., Strachan, D. *et al.* (1993). Self-reported prevalence of asthma symptoms in children in Australia, England, Germany and New Zealand: an international comparison using the ISAAC protocol. *European Respiratory Journal*, **6**, 1455–61.

Peat, J. K., van den Berg, R. H., Green, W. F., Mellis, C. M., Leeder, S. R., and Woolcock, A. J. (1994). Changing prevalence of asthma in Australian children. *British Medical Journal*, **308**, 1591–6.

Scottish Intercollegiate Guidelines Network. (1996). *Obesity in Scotland. Integrating prevention with weight management* (Pilot edn), pp. 10–11. SIGN, Glasgow University.

Seaton, A., Godden, D. J., and Brown, K. (1994). Increase in asthma; a more toxic environment or a more susceptible population. *Thorax*, **49**, 172–4.

Seidell, J. C., de Groot, L. C. P. G. M., van Sonsberg, J. L. A., Deurenberg, P., and Hautvast, J. G. A. J. (1986). Associations of moderate and severe overweight with self-reported illness and medical care in Dutch adults. *American Journal of Public Health*, **76**, 264–9.

Serdula, M. K., Ivery, D., Coates, R. J., Freedman, D. S. Williamson, D. F., and Byers, T. (1993). Do obese children become obese adults? A review of the literature. *Preventive Medicine*, **22**, 167–77.

Shaheen, S. O., Sterne, J. A. C., Tucker, J. S., and Florey, C. du V. (1998). Birth weight, childhood lower respiratory tract infection, and adult lung function. *Thorax*, **53**, 549–53.

Shaheen, S. O., Sterne, J. A. C., Montgomery, S. M., and Azima, H. (1999). Birthweight, body mass index and asthma in young adults. *Thorax*, **54**, 386–402.

Shepherd, J., Betteridge, D. J., Durrington, P., Laker, M., Lewis, B., Mann, J., *et al.* (1987). Strategies for reducing coronary heart disease and desirable limits for blood lipid concentrations: guidelines of the British Hyperlipidaemia Association. *British Medical Journal*, **295**, 1245–6.

Smith, A. M., Chinn, S., and Rona, R. J. (1980). Social factors and height gain of primary schoolchildren in England and Scotland. *Annals of Human Biology*, **7**, 115–24.

Somerville, S. M. and Rona, R. J. (1993). Respiratory conditions, including asthma, and height in primary school. *Annals of Human Biology*, **20**, 369–80.

Somerville, S. M., Rona, R. J., and Chinn, S. (1984). Obesity and respiratory symptoms in primary school. *Archives of Disease in Childhood*, **59**, 940–4.

Somerville, S. M., Rona, R. J., and Chinn, S. (1988). Passive smoking and respiratory conditions in primary school children. *Journal of Epidemiology and Community Health*, **42**, 105–10.

Somerville, S. M., Rona, R. J., Chinn, S., and Qureshi, S. (1996). Family credit and uptake of school meals in primary school. *Journal of Public Health Medicine*, **18**, 98–106.

Sorensen, T. I. A. and Price, R. A. (1990). Secular trends in body mass index among Danish young men. *International Journal of Obesity*, **14**, 411–19.

Speight, A. N. P., Lee, D. A., and Hey, E. N. (1983). Underdiagnosis and undertreatment of asthma in childhood. *British Medical Journal*, **286**, 1253–6.

Speizer, F. E., Ferris, B., Bishop, Y. M., and Spengler, J. (1980). Respiratory disease rates and pulmonary function in children associated with NO2 exposure. *American Review of Respiratory Disease*, **121**, 3–10.

Sporik, R., Holgate, S. T., Platts-Mills, T. A. E., and Cogswell, J. J. (1990). Exposure to house dust mite allergen (Der p 1) and the development of asthma in childhood. A prospective study. *New England Journal of Medicine*, **323**, 502–7.

Sporik, R., Johnstone, J. H., and Cogswell, J. J. (1991). Longitudinal study of cholesterol values in 68 children from birth to 11 years of age. *Archives of Disease in Childhood*, **66**, 134–7.

Stenberg, A. and Läckgren, G. (1994). Desmopressin tablets in the treatment of severe nocturnal enuresis in adolescents. *Pediatrics*, **94**, 841–6.

Stern, M. and Walker, W. A. (1985). Food allergy and intolerance. *Pediatric Clinics of North America*, **32**, 471–92.

Strachan, D. P. (1989). Hay fever, hygiene, and household size. *British Medical Journal*, **299**, 1259–60.

Strachan, D. P. (1997). Allergy and family size: a riddle worth solving. *Clinical and Experimental Allergy*, **27**, 235–7.

Strachan, D. P., Anderson, H. R., Limb, E. S., O'Neill, A., and Wells, N. (1994). A national survey of asthma prevalence and treatment in Great Britain. *Archives of Disease in Childhood*, **70**, 174–8.

Stunkard, A. J., Harris, J. R., Pedersen, L. P., and McClearn, G. E. (1990). The body-mass index of twins who have been reared apart. *The New England Journal of Medicine*, **322**, 1483–7.

Szklo, M. (1979). Epidemiological patterns of blood pressure in children. *Epidemiological Reviews*, **1**, 143–69.

Tager, I. B., Weiss, S. T., Munoz, A., Rosner, B., and Speizer, F. E. (1983). Longitudinal study of the effects of maternal smoking on pulmonary function in children. *New England Journal of Medicine*, **309**, 699–703.

Tager, I. B., Segal, M. R., Munoz, A., Weiss, S. T., and Speizer, F. E. (1987). The effect of maternal cigarette smoking on the pulmonary function of children and adolescents. Analyses of data from two populations. *American Review of Respiratory Disease*, **136**, 1366–70.

Takahashi, Y., Kipnis, D. M., and Daughaday, W. H. (1968). Growth hormone secretion during sleep. *Journal of Clinical Investigation*, **47**, 2079–90.

Tanner, J. M. (1951). Some notes on the reporting of growth data. *Human Biology*, **23**, 93–159.

Tanner, J. M. (1981). *A history of the study of human growth*, pp. 142, 299–379, 381–94. Cambridge University Press, Cambridge.

Tanner, J. M. (1986). Growth as a mirror of conditions of society: secular trends and class distinctions. In *Human growth: a multidisciplinary review* (ed. A. Demirjian), pp. 3–34. Taylor and Francis, London.

Tanner, J. M. and Whitehouse, R. H. (1962). Standards for subcutaneous fat in British children. Percentiles for thickness of skinfolds over triceps and below scapula. *British Medical Journal*, **1**, 446–50.

Tanner, J. M., Whitehouse, R. H., and Takaishi, M. (1966). Standards from birth to maturity for height, weight, height velocity, and weight velocity: British children, 1965 Parts I and II. *Archives of Disease in Childhood*, **41**, 454–71, 613–35.

Taylor, B., Wadsworth, J., Wadsworth, M., and Peckham, C. (1984). Changes in the reported prevalence of childhood eczema since the 1939–45 war. *Lancet*, **ii**, 1255–7.

Thompson, S. and Rey, J. M. (1995). Functional enuresis: is desmopressin the answer? *Journal of the American Academy of Child and Adolescent Psychiatry*, **34**, 266–71.

Topp, S. G., Cook, J., Holland, W. W., and Elliott, A. (1970). Influence of environmental factors on height and weight of schoolchildren. *British Journal of Preventive and Social Medicine*, **24**, 154–62.

Topp, S. G., Cook, J., and Elliott A. (1972). Measurement of nutritional intake among schoolchildren: aspects of methodology. *British Journal of Preventive and Social Medicine*, **26**, 106–11.

Townsend, P., Phillimore, P., and Beattie, A. (1988). *Health and deprivation. Inequalities and the North*, pp. 34–8. Routledge, London.

Troiano, R. P., Flegal, K. M., Kuczmarski, R. J., Campbell, S. M., and Johnson, C. L. (1995). Overweight prevalence and trends for children and adolescents. *Archives of Pediatric and Adolescent Medicine*, **149**, 1085–91.

Vela-Bueno, A., Bixler, E. O., Dobladez-Blanco, B., Rubio, M. E., Mathison, R. E., and Kales, A. (1985). Prevalence in night terrors and nightmares in elementary school children: a pilot study. *Research in Community Psychology and Psychiatric Behaviour*, **10**, 177–88.

Vignerová, J. and Bláha, P. (1998). The growth of the Czech children during the past 40 years. In: *Secular growth changes in Europe* (ed. É. B. Bodzsar and C. Susanne), pp. 93–107. Eövös Loránd University Press, Budapest.

Volkmer, R. E., Ruffin, R., Wigg, N. R., and Davies, N. (1995). The prevalence of respiratory symptoms in South Australian pre-school children: II factors associated with indoor air quality. *Journal of Paediatric Child Health*, **31**, 116–20.

von Mutius E., Martinez, F. D., Fritzsch, C., Nicolai, C., Reitmeir, P., and Thiemann, H-H. (1994). Skin test reactivity and number of siblings. *British Medical Journal*, **308**, 692–5.

Voss, L. D. (1995). Can we measure growth? *Journal of Medical Screening*, **2**, 164–7.

Ware, J. H., Dockery, D. W., Spiro, A., Speizer, F. E., and Ferris, B. G. (1984). Passive smoking, gas cooking, and respiratory health of children living in six cities. *American Review of Respiratory Disease*, **129**, 366–74.

Warner, J. O., Gotz, M., Landau, L. I., Levison, H., Milner, A. D., Pedersen, S., *et al.* (1989). Management of asthma: a consensus statement. *Archives of Disease in Childhood*, **64**, 1065–79.

Warzak, W. J. (1993). Psychosocial implications of nocturnal enuresis. *Clinical Pediatrics Special Edition*, 38–40.

Webber, L. S., Harsha, D. W., Phillips, G. T., Srinavasan, S. R., Simpson, J. W., and Berenson, G. S. (1991). Cardiovascular risk factors in hispanic, white, and black children: the Brooks County heart study. *American Journal of Epidemiology*, **133**, 704–14.

Webber, L. S., Wattigney, W. A., Srinivasan, S. R., and Berenson, G. S. (1995). Obesity studies in Bogolusa. *American Journal of Medical Sciences*, **310** (Suppl. 1), S53–61.

Weiss, S. T. (1997). Diet as a risk factor for asthma. In *The rising trends in asthma*. Ciba Foundation Symposium 206, pp. 244–53. Wiley, Chichester.

Whincup, P. H., Cook, D. G., and Shaper, A. G. (1989). Early influences on blood pressure: a study of school children aged 5–7 years. *British Medical Journal*. **299**, 587–91.

Whincup, P. H., Cook, D. G., Papacosta, O., and Walker, M. (1992). Childhood blood pressure, body build, and birthweight: geographical associations with cardiovascular mortality. *Journal of Epidemiology and Community Health*, **46**, 396–402.

White, A., Nicolaas, G., Foster, K., Browne F., and Carey, S. (ed.) (1993). *Health survey for England 1991*, pp. 41, 48–50. HMSO, London.

Widdowson, E. M. (1951). Mental contentment and physical growth. *Lancet*, **i**, 1316.

Widdowson, E. M. and McCance, R. A. (1954). Studies on the nutritive value of bread and on the effect of variations in the extraction rate of flour on the growth of undernourished children. Medical Research Council, Special Report Series, No. 287. HMSO, London.

Willetts W. C. (1990). Food frequency methods. *Nutritional epidemiology*, Chapter 5, pp. 69–91. Oxford University Press, Oxford.

Wilson, R. S. (1979). Twin growth: initial deficit, recovery, and trends in concordance from birth to nine years. *Annals of Human Biology*, **6**, 93–105.

Wissow, L. S., Gittelsohn, A. M., Szklo, M., Starfield, M., and Mussman, M. (1988). Poverty, race, and hospitalization for childhood asthma. *American Journal of Public Health*, **78**, 777–82.

Woolson, R. F. and Clarke, W. R. (1984). Analysis of categorical incomplete data. *Journal of the Royal Statistical Society A*, **147**, 87–99.

Yip, R., Scanlon, K., and Trowbridge, F. (1993). Trends patterns in height and weight status of low-income US children. *Critical Reviews in Food Science and Nutrition*, **33**, 409–21.

Young, E., Patel, S., Stoneham, M. D., Rona, R. J., and Wilkinson, J. D. (1987). The prevalence of reactions to food additives in a survey population. *Journal of the Royal College of Physicians, London*, **78**, 5–11.

Young, E., Stoneham, M. D., Petruckevitch, A., Barton, J., and Rona, R. (1994). A population study of food intolerance. *Lancet*, **343**, 1127–30.

Zeger, S. L. and Liang, K-Y. (1986). Longitudinal data analysis for discrete and continuous outcomes. *Biometrics*, **42**, 121–30.

Zetterstrom, O., Osterman, K., Machado, L., and Johansson, S. G. O. (1981). Another smoking hazard: raised serum IgE concentration and increased risk of occupational allergy. *British Medical Journal*, **283**, 1215–17.

Index

abnormal results, communication to parents and doctors 25–6
'Administration manual' 23
administration of long-term large studies 26
  activities related to study 23–4
  communicating abnormal results to parents and doctors 25–6
  fieldwork 24–5
  parental consent 25
  parents' comments 26
  requirements 21
  team and network of collaborators 21–2
administrator 22
Afro-Caribbean children
  auxological perspective 106
  blood pressure 61
  cholesterol 60
  disturbed sleep 88, 90
  enuresis, nocturnal 86, 9
  height 32, 44, 46
  obesity 40–1, 54, 55, 57
  respiratory illness and lung function 65, 66, 71
air pollution 64, 98–9
allergens, exposure to 81
allergic conditions 81
  see also asthma
antibiotics for asthma 72
anti-inflammatory agents for asthma 72
antitussives for asthma 72
asthma
  community management 71–2
  ethnicity 65, 66
  family size and poverty 69–71
  height 48, 67–8
  obesity 57, 68, 70, 82
  secular trends 82, 99
    background 79
    first report and replication of findings 79–82
  smoking, parental 77
atopy, clinical 88
auxological perspective of NSHG
  achievement 102–3

background 101–2
  fatness, measurement of 105–6
  secular changes and dynamics of heredity–environment interaction 106–7
  surveys vs. surveillance 103–5

background to study 1
  birth of NSHG 2–4
  historical perspective 1–2
Bentham, Jeremy 101
β_2 agonists for asthma 72
biceps skinfold thickness 12, 50, 56
bioelectrical impedance analysis (BIA) 51
birth order
  asthma 69, 70
  disturbed sleep 88
  enuresis, nocturnal 86
birthweight
  blood pressure 60, 61
  height 33, 45, 46
  obesity 51, 52, 53, 56, 57
  respiratory illness and lung function 68
blood pressure
  abnormal results 26
  coronary heart disease 58, 60–3
  obesity 56, 57
body mass index (BMI) 17, 35
  Health Survey for England 42
  parental 41, 51, 52–3, 56, 57
boys
  cholesterol 59, 60
  enuresis, nocturnal 86, 87
  height 101, 102, 104
    secular trend 28, 29–30, 31–2
  obesity 35–6, 37–9, 40–1
  respiratory illness and lung function 66
    asthma 79–80
    parental smoking 74, 75, 76
bronchial responsiveness (BHR) 65–6
bronchitis
  obesity 57, 68
  secular trend 79–80, 81
  smoking, parental 75, 77
bronchodilators for asthma 71–2

Thatcher, Margaret 1, 98
Thompson, Professor Angus 3–4
total body water (TBW) 51
Townsend deprivation score 70
translation of letters and questionnaires 13, 23
trend calculation using mixed longitudinal data
    measurements 17–18
    respiratory symptoms 18
triceps skinfold thickness
    birth of NSHG 3
    blood pressure 62
    calculation of trends 18
    measurement 12
        quality control 14–15
    obesity 50, 51, 52, 54, 56–7
        secular trend 35, 36, 38–42
    respiratory illness 68
    standard deviation score 16, 17

undernutrition 2, 43
unemployment 33, 46, 48
United States of America 33–4, 42
University of London Computing Centre
    (ULCC) 15–16
Urdu children
    blood pressure 61
    cholesterol 59, 60
    height 32, 44, 48
    obesity 40–1, 55, 56

vegetarians 48
venepuncture 58
    ethical issues 25

verification of data 15

weight
    birth of NSHG 3
    calculation of trends 18
    historical perspective 1
    measurement 12
        quality control 14
    obesity, secular trend in 35
    respiratory illness 68
    standard deviation score 16, 17
weight-for-height
    auxological perspective 106
    birth of NSHG 3
    blood pressure 60, 61, 62
    calculation of trends 18
    coronary heart disease 62
    obesity 50, 51–2, 56–7
        secular trend 35–7, 39, 40, 41–2
    respiratory illness 68
    standard deviation score 16, 17
wheeze
    community management 71–2
    disturbed sleep 88, 90
    ethnicity 65, 66
    family size and poverty 69, 70, 71
    height 48, 49, 67
    length of gestation 68
    obesity 57, 68
    secular trend 79–80, 81, 82
    smoking, parental 75–7
Wilberforce, William 101
World War II 1